Erythrocytes as Drug Carriers in Medicine

Erythrocytes as Drug Carriers in Medicine

Edited by

Ulrich Sprandel
Kreiskrankenhaus
Marktoberdorf, Germany

and

James L. Way
Texas A&M University
College Station, Texas

Springer Science+Business Media, LLC

Library of Congress Cataloging-in-Publication Data

On file

Proceedings of the Sixth Meeting of the International Society for the Use of Resealed Erythrocytes, held July 25 – 28, 1996, in Irsee, Germany

DOI 10.1007/978-1-4899-0044-9

Originally published by Plenum Press, New York in 1997

MyCopy version of the original edition 1997

10 9 8 7 6 5 4 3 2 1

PREFACE

The sixth meeting on the use of resealed annealed red blood cells was held in Irsee, Germany by the International Society for the Use of Resealed Erythrocytes (ISURE) on July 25–28, 1996. Although earlier meetings focused on the technology toward development of methods and standardization for efficient, consistent encapsulation, most of the present studies now are directed toward the application use of these carrier blood cells. Basic studies now have been directed toward exploration of commercial applications. Indeed, clinical trials were initiated to evaluate the dose-response curves employing L-asparagenase in human patients. Also, studies have shown the use of thrombolytic agent in erythrocyte carriers with the use of human red blood cells to provide a new conceptual approach in thrombolytic therapy to prevent thrombosis in individuals with higher risk factors. For example, with the use of carrier red blood cells, the thrombolytic agents will have a greater potential of acting on clot formation without systemic activation and thus lower the risk of hemorrhage, which is always prevalent in the thrombolytic therapy. Erythrocyte carrier systems are still quite unique and useful as specific targeting agents with a prolonged, sustained action with minimal immunologic or other toxic effects. The stability of this carrier system provides greater applications, especially of enzymes and proteins, by minimizing immunologic reactions and enhancing stability. Each of these studies are directed to minimize the toxicity so that higher doses such as IL2 can be used and it permits the use of more toxic prodrugs such as 3′-azidothymidine homodinucleotide as an anti-HIV drug. The focus of erythrocyte carriers now appears to be in the area of applications—especially, commercial area, which is the logical sequence as this area of endeavors matures.

CONTENTS

1

A MODEL FOR THE ASSESSMENT OF HUMAN RECOMBINANT INTERLEUKIN 2 (RIL2) COATED ERYTHROCYTES AS A DELIVERY SYSTEM FOR IMMUNOTHERAPY

R. B. Moyes and J. R. DeLoach

USDA-ARS-FAPRL
College Station, Texas, 77845

1. ABSTRACT

A carrier system for IL2 is needed in order to circumvent the toxicity associated with high dose interleukin 2 (IL2) administration and its rapid clearance from circulation. Erythrocytes (RBC) coated with recombinant interleukin 2 (rIL2) provide a means of delivering IL2 into the system in a continuous, low dose manner which in turn maintains a low, potentially non-toxic, IL2 concentration. Murine RBC coated with rIL2 (RBC-rIL2) induce cytotoxicity (21–31%) upon cytotoxic testing of spleens cells stimulated *in vivo*. Using the murine Meth A sarcoma model, the effectiveness of this RBC-rIL2 vehicle is demonstrated *in vivo* by a 84% reduction in tumor size as compared to the soluble rIL2 treated mice. Moreover, the RBC-rIL2 vehicle is able to induce tumoricidal cytotoxicity with very low rIL2 concentrations (about 10,000 I.U. of rIL2 per mouse). These results indicate that rIL2 retains its biological activity when bound to the RBC and therefore could prove useful as a therapeutic delivery system for cancer treatment.

2. INTRODUCTION

Interleukin 2 (IL2), a lymphocytotrophic hormone secreted exclusively by stimulated T cells, has been characterized to be of major importance in both cell mediated and humoral immunity. IL2 acts on several different cell types including natural killer (NK) cells, B cells, and T cells resulting in cellular proliferation and augmentation of their immunological functions. In the case of NK cells, both secretory and cytolytic capabilities are markedly enhanced. NK cells release a repertoire of cytokines as a result of IL2 introduction including interferon gamma (IFN-γ), granulocyte-macrophage colony stimulating factor (GM-CSF), and tumor necrosis factor (TNF-α,β)(Ritz 1988, Kaplan 1992), all which in turn stimulate monocyte and

Erythrocytes as Drug Carriers in Medicine, edited by Sprandel and Way
Plenum Press, New York, 1997

macrophage responses. Thus IL2, in concert with an array of stimulated cells and lymphokines, is an important immunological defense against infection and tumorigenic growth.

Lymphokine therapy, especially IL2 therapy, is being used experimentally in high dose regimes to treat cancer (Lotze 1986, Rosenberg 1987). These clinical tests have shown that IL2 administration can mediate the regression of established tumors especially renal cell carcinoma and malginant melanoma (Sosman 1993) in both experimental animal models and humans. However, high dose IL2 immunotherapy is toxic to the patient resulting in capillary leak syndrome due to the release of other cytokines, most notably TNF-α, eventually leading to hypotension (Mier 1990).

It is difficult to maintain plasma IL2 levels due to the rapid clearance of IL2 from circulation. It has been previously shown that, regardless of route of injection, by two hours post injection, no IL2 activity is detectable in the serum (Cheever 1986). Anti- tumor effects of IL2 correlate more strongly with low sustained IL2 plasma levels than with intermittent peak IL2 plasma levels (Cheever 1985). Therefore, any method that sustains delivery of IL2 at a low constant level would circumvent high dose toxicity and at the same time probably increase the therapeutic index of IL2.

The purpose of this investigation was to observe the biological effects produced by IL2-coated erythrocytes both *in vitro* and *in vivo* in the murine system.

3. MATERIALS AND METHODS

3.1. Media

RPMI 1640 (JRH Biosciences, Lenexa,KS) was supplemented with 2mM L-glutamine (Sigma, St. Louis, MO), and 5% Antimycotic/Antibiotic solution (Sigma) in all cases, and with 10% fetal bovine serum (FBS)(JRH Biosciences) (RPMI-FBS) for cell culture.

3.2. Cell Lines

The WEHI 164 cell line, a fibrosarcoma originally induced by subcutaneous injection of 3-methylcholanthrene in Balb/c mice (ATCC CRL 1751, Rockville, MD) served as a syngeneic tumor line for *in vivo* tumor studies. The malignant murine cell line, YAC-1 (ATCC TIB 160) was used in the *in vitro* cytotoxicity assays. Both cell lines were maintained in culture in RPMI-FBS. An IL2-dependent cytotoxic T cell line, CTLL (ATCC TIB 214) was maintained on RPMI-FBS with the addition of T-stim (Collaborative Biomedical Products, Bedford, MA), an IL2 supplement.

3.3. Cytokines

Recombinant human interleukin 2 (rIL2) was purchased from Cellular Products (Buffalo, NY; supplied by Cetus Corporation). Each vial contained 100ug of rIL2 (15.4 kD) and was stabilized in a 2% FBS solution.

3.4. Mice

Mouse spleens were obtained from female Balb/c mice which had been purchased from Harlan Laboratories (Houston, Texas). The mice were housed and fed ad libitum according to the USDA guidelines established by the Animal Care and Use Committee.

3.5. Mitogens

Phytohemagglutin P (PHA) and lipopolysaccharide (LPS) were both obtained from Sigma and used at a concentration of 1ug/well in Falcon 96 well plates (Baxter Scientific Products) or 1ug/ml when added to tissue culture flasks.

3.6. Isolation of Erythrocytes

Mice were anesthetized with CO_2 and blood was collected via cardiac puncture. The RBC were washed 3 times with a PBS buffer containing 10 mM glucose, 4 mM $MgCl_2$, 5 mM adenosine, and 5 mM inosine (Sigma) (complete buffer referred to as MBA) at 400 x g at 4°C for 10 minutes. The buffy coat was removed and discarded after the first wash. Erythrocytes were counted using a computerized Coulter counter (Hileah, FL) and were resuspended in MBA to a concentration of 10^{10} cells per ml.

3.7. Adsorption of IL2 to Erythrocytes

RBC were resuspended in sterile eppendorf tubes (USA Scientific, Ocala, FL) to 10^{10} cells per ml and incubated with rIL2 at a ratio of 72,000 I.U./10^9 erythrocytes (unless otherwise stated) with gentle rotation for 30 min at 4°C. The cells were then washed 3 times with 4 volumes of MBA. This technique yielded approximately 8000–12,000 I.U. of rIL2 coated on the surface per 10^9 erythrocytes as determined by the CTLL bioassay.

3.8. *In Vitro* Cytotoxicity Assay

For radiolabeling of the target cells, YAC-1 mouse myeloma cells were suspended to 10^7 cells/ml of RPMI-FBS and incubated with 100 ul/ml of ^{51}Chromium (200–900 Ci/g, ICN Radiochemicals, Irvine, CA) at 37°C for 120 minutes. The target cells were washed 3 times, diluted to a concentration of 10^6 cells/ml, and dispensed at 100 ul per well in Falcon 96 well U bottom microtiter plates (Baxter Scientific Products). One hundred ul of the spleen cells at final effector: target ratio of 25:1 were then dispensed in the microtiter plate. Background or spontaneous release was determined by incubating labeled target cells in RPMI-FBS alone, and total release was determined by incubating labeled target cells in 100 ul of 1% sodium dodecyl sulfate (Biorad, Richmond, CA) solution. Plates were centrifuged at 900 rpm for 5 minutes and then incubated for 24 hr in a 5% CO_2 incubator. After incubation, the plates were again centrifuged and 150 ul from each well was collected and counted in a LKB 1282 Compugamma gamma counter (Gaithersburg, MD). Cytotoxicity was quantitated as follows:

$$\%\,\text{of specific Cr release} = \frac{\text{experimental release cpm} - \text{spontaneous release cpm} \times 100}{\text{total release cpm} - \text{spontaneous release cpm}}$$

3.9. *In Vivo* Activation

Balb/c mice were injected i.p. with 100 ul of one of the following preparations: normal RBC (10^9RBC/mouse), RBC-rIL2 (10^9 RBC + 8000–12,000 I.U. IL2/mouse), soluble rIL2 (72,000 IU/mouse), or MBA (100ul/mouse), unless otherwise indicated. Depending on the experiment, mice received either 1 to 4 injections at one injection per week, or 4 injections at 3 injections per week (Friday, Monday, Wednesday, Friday). Spleens were harvested 4 days after the last injection.

3.10. Cytokine Determination

IFN-γ production was determined using a commercial ELISA kit (Genzyme, Cambridge, MA). The kit had a sensitivity level of 125 pg IFN-γ/ml and had no detectable cross-reaction with mouse IL1-α, IL2, IL3, IL4, or TNF-α. TNF production was analyzed using the Genzyme TNF ELISA kit which had a sensitivity level of 100 pg/ml and did not cross-react with IL1-α, IL2, IL3, GM-CSF, or IFN-γ (according to the manufacturer).

3.11. Bioassay of Erythrocyte-Bound rIL2

RBC-rIL2 at 10^{10} cells/ml were carried through 3 freeze/ thaw cycles to assure complete lysis of the RBC. Dilutions in complete media were made and 50 ul of each dilution were added to 100 ul of CTLL cells (10^5 cells/ml) in a 96 well flat bottom plate and incubated for 20 hours at 37°C in 5% CO_2 and then pulsed with 0.1 uCi/well of [^{3}H]thymidine (ICN, Irvine CA) for the final 4 hours. Cells were harvested using a Skatron cell harvester (Sterling, VA) onto glass fiber filters and [^{3}H]thymidine incorporation was determined by liquid scintillation counting. Normal RBC were lysed and used as control supernatants and rIL2 standards were used to construct calibration curves for assessing IL2 levels in the RBC-rIL2 samples.

3.12. Pharmacokinetics of RBC-rIL2

Erythrocytes were labeled with Cr^{51} in order to follow their survival in circulation. Cells were resuspended to 10^{10} cells/ml in MBA and were mixed with 100 ul of $Na_2{}^{51}CrO_4$ (1mCi/ml) for 30 min at 37°C followed by a wash in MBA/0.1% BSA then two washes in MBA. Cells were then incubated with rIL2 as indicated above. Balb/c mice (5 per group) were injected i.p. with 100 ul of chromium labeled normal RBC or RBC-rIL2. Blood was drawn via cardiac puncture at time 0, 24, 48, and 72 hours. Ten microliters of whole blood was counted in triplicate in a LKB 1282 Compugamma gamma counter.

3.13. Antitumor Efficacy

On day 1, Balb/c mice were injected subcutaneously (s.c.) in the left flank with 1 x 10^5 cells/100ul of syngeneic WEHI 164 tumor cells. On days 1, 8, 15, and 22 the mice were injected i.p. with 100ul of RBC-rIL2, normal RBC, soluble rIL2, or MBA all prepared as described above. On day 29, the tumors were excised and weighed and spleens harvested for further *in vitro* testing. Single cell suspensions of the spleen cells were prepared as described above. Cells were dispensed in 24 well plates at 20 x 10^6 cells/2 ml RPMI-FBS/well and 25 ul of PHA (100ug/ml) was added to each well. Supernatants were harvested at 24, 48, and 72 hr and assayed for the presence of cytokines.

3.14. Statistical Analyses

For cytokine release assays and significance of treatment effects, the student's T test was performed using the MicroCal Origin Software Package (Northampton, MA).

4. RESULTS

4.1. *In Vivo* Induction of Cytotoxic Activity

It was of interest to determine what immunological effects RBC-rIL2 had *in vivo*. Table 1 shows the results of several representative experiments of mice injected i.p. as indicated with RBC ± rIL2. Only the mice receiving RBC-rIL2 showed any increases in *in vitro* cytotoxicity above background controls. Spleen cells from mice injected with 72,000 I.U. of soluble rIL2 (6–8 times greater rIL2 concentration than the injection of 10^9 RBC-rIL2), and spleen cells from mice injected with control RBC demonstrated no increase in the level of cytotoxicity above background controls. It should be noted, however, that with increased injections per week, normal RBC appear to begin to have a slight effect on the cytotoxic potential.

4.2. *In Vivo* Interferon Gamma Production

Serum and spleen cells were collected from mice injected i.p. with RBC±rIL2. Based upon ELISA testing of the serum samples from both sets of mice, no IFN-γ could be detected. However, if spleen cells from both groups were incubated with LPS for 24 hr *in vitro* and the supernatants were again tested, appreciable amounts of IFN-γ could be detected in the mice that had originally been injected with RBC-rIL2 (Figure 1). These results indicated that the presence of rIL2 as presented by or released from the surface of the RBC was having an effect on the immune system, and this effect became evident upon *in vitro* culture.

Table 1. *In vivo* activation of Balb/c spleen cells with rIL2 coated RBC for *in vitro* cytotoxicity against YAC-1 tumor cells

I.P. Injection	No. of injections	Injections per week	% Cytotoxicity by spleen cells against YAC-1 cells*
RBC-IL2^			
2 x 10^7	1	1	30.9±2.6[a,b]
1 x 10^9	4	1	21.1±2.1[a,b]
1 x 10^9	4	3	30.6±0.2[a,b]
normal RBC			
2 x 10^7	1	1	1.6±0.3
1 x 10^9	4	1	0.3±0.2
1 x 10^9	4	3	17.4±0.5[a]
soluble rIL2			
72,000 I.U.	4	1	11.5±0.7
72,000 I.U.	4	3	6.7±2.2

*Balb/c mice were injected i.p. and spleens were harvested 4 days after the last injection and used in an *in vitro* cytotoxicity assay against YAC-1 tumor cells. Results expressed as the % cytotoxicity; mean ±sem 8 mice/group.

^8000-12,000 I.U. of rIL2 per 10^9 RBC.

[a]$P<0.001$ compared to cytotoxic activity of spleen cells stimulated with soluble rIL2.

[b]$P<0.001$ compared to cytotoxic activity of mice injected with RBC using the same treatment schedule.

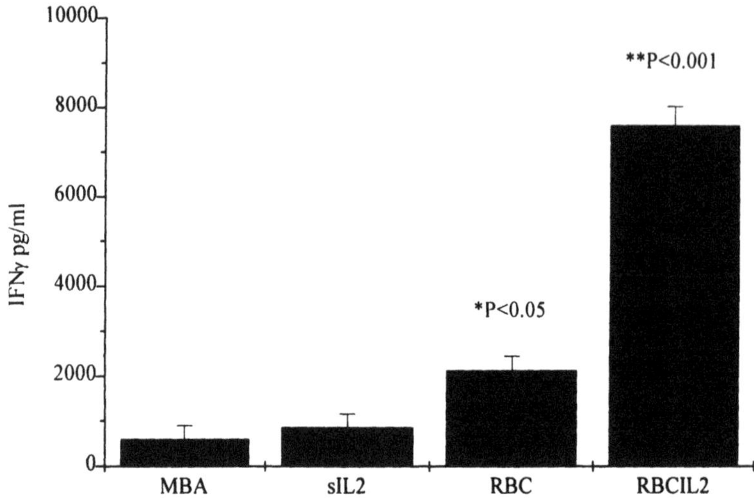

Figure 1. Interferon gamma production by Balb/c spleen cells after *in vivo* stimulation by RBC ± rIL2. Mice were injected i.p. with RBC ± rIL2 (100 ul of 10^{10} RBC/ml), 100 ul MBA, or 45,000 I.U. rIL2 on Friday, Monday, Wednesday, and Friday and then the spleens were harvested on the following Tuesday. Spleen cells were incubated at a concentration of 100 x 10^6 cells/10 mls RPMI + 10% FBS /25cm^2 flask with 100 ul of LPS (1ug/ml) for 24 hours. Supernatants were tested for the presence of IFN-γ. *P<0.05 versus soluble rIL2 results. **P<0.001 compared to the RBC control.

4.3. Pharmacokinetics of Chromium 51 Labeled RBC

When washed RBC from RBC-rIL2 and RBC injected mice were tested for the presence of chromium labeled cells, 60–65% of normal RBC and RBC-rIL2 were still in circulation at 72 hr (Figure 2). There was no significant difference in the numbers between the two treatment groups. Plasma rIL2 concentrations from these two groups of mice were too low to detect with the bioassay due to the initial low concentration of rIL2 injected. However, bioassay of *in vitro* samples of RBC-rIL2 incubated at 37°C in RPMI-FBS demonstrated the presence of rIL2 on the RBC through the 72 hr tested (a normal RBC culture was run in parallel as a control , data not shown).

4.4. Antitumor Effect of RBC-rIL2 Vehicle

After 4 injections of RBC-rIL2, normal RBC, soluble rIL2, or MBA in Meth A tumor bearing mice, an 84% reduction of tumor growth was apparent in the RBC-rIL2 injected animals (Figure 3). No significant difference in tumor weights were found between the other three treatment groups.

4.5. Cytokine Production of Cells from Tumor Bearing Mice

Spleen cells from Meth A tumor bearing mice which had been injected with the various treatment groups, were cultured *in vitro* and the supernatants were tested for cytokine production (Figure 4). The cells from the RBC injected group produced significantly

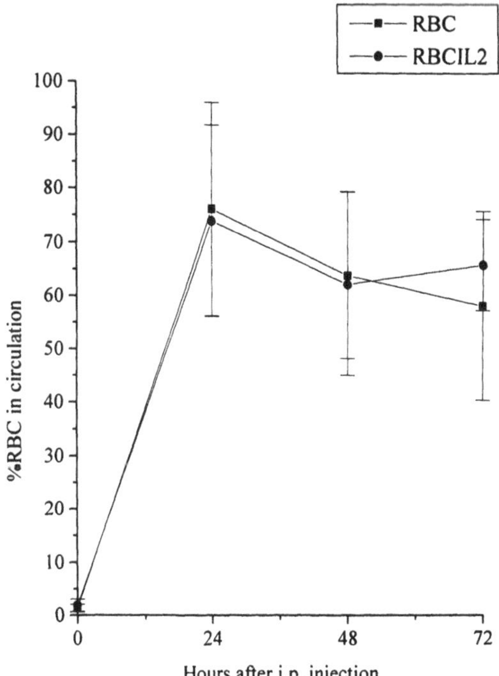

Figure 2. Pharmacokinetics of normal RBC and RBC-rIL2 which were chromium 51 labeled and injected i.p. in Balb/c mice. Samples were taken at 0, 24, 48, and 72 hr and 10 ul was counted in triplicate. Graph is representative of 3 experiments with 5 mice per time point per experiment.

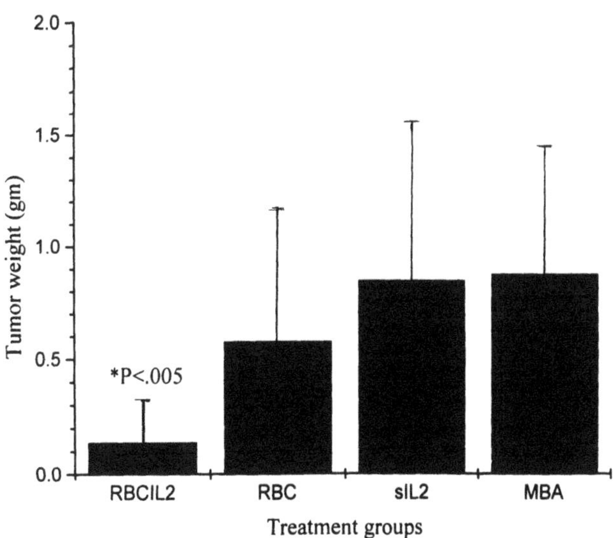

Figure 3. Balb/c mice bearing syngeneic Meth A tumors (inoculated s.c.) were treated with 100 ul i.p. of RBC-rIL2, normal RBC, soluble rIL2, or MBA once a week for 4 weeks. On week 5, tumors were harvested and weighed. The tumors were significantly reduced in the RBC-rIL2 treatment group only.

higher levels of IFN-γ and TNF than the three other treatment groups. However, the RBC-rIL2 treated group also produced significant amounts of IFN-γ as compared to the soluble rIL2 and MBA treated mice.

5. DISCUSSION

Several laboratories have used various IL2 preparations in order to extend the serum half-life of IL2 (Johnston 1992, Crum 1991, Thrombe 1984, Poste 1979, Anderson 1992). The use of RBC offers several advantages over previously described techniques. These advantages include the following: 1) RBC-IL2 preparations are ready for use after a simple 30 minute incubation period at 4°C with washed RBC and rIL2. 2) RBC are natural biological products so no chemicals are introduced into the body. 3) RBC-rIL2 preparations can be injected by any route, and previous studies (DeLoach 1986) have shown that RBC injected either i.p. or i.v. have the same half-life in circulation. 4) The use of RBC allows the biological agent of interest to either be encapsulated within or bound to the surface of the RBC. 5) RBC can be utilized as a targeting system for diffusible molecules (Ropars 1987). Intraperitoneal injection allows for extravascular targeting of RBC to peritoneal macrophages (DeLoach 1986), and pretreatment of RBC with glutaraldehyde targets the RBC to the liver (DeLoach 1983). Chiarantini et al.(1992) have coupled Thy1 antibody to the surface of the RBC to signal formation of rosettes with CTLL cells. Thus, with the aid of specific antibodies, RBC can be directed toward any area of interest within the body. 6) RBC also express natural receptors on their surface which can be exploited for the purpose of immunotherapy. For example, human RBC express 1772–3290 copies of CD58

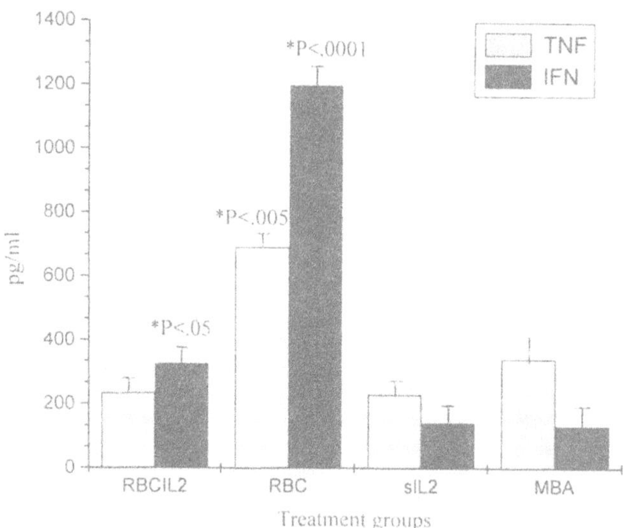

Figure 4. Spleen cell suspensions were made from the spleens of the mice used in the Figure 4 experiment. The cells were cultured at 20 x 10^6 cells/2 mls with 25 ul of PHA for 24, 48, and 72 hr (separate wells were harvested in triplicate per time period). The IFN-γ results are from 24 hr supernatants and the TNF-α results are from 72 hr culture supernatants for optimum cytokine production.

(LFA-3) per RBC (Anstee 1991) which is the natural ligand for CD2. The presence of LFA-3 could account for the natural immunostimulatory or adjuvant effect often associated with RBC. 7) RBC-rIL2 injection maintains a much longer serum half-life than bolus rIL2 injection, so the need for frequent or daily injections or catheterization, which increases the risk of infection is avoided. 8) A patient's own RBC are used for coating of the rIL2 so no new problems associated with introduced chemicals or foreign blood are encountered. 9) The concentration of rIL2 on the RBC-rIL2 vehicle is a low concentration thus circumventing the problems associated with high dose toxicity. 10) An added benefit is the fact that RBC can exert an adjuvant effect, so even less of the rIL2 would be required for treatment.

In vivo, RBC-rIL2 generated 21–31% cytotoxicity as compared to 0–17% induced by i.p. injection of normal RBC. Soluble rIL2, even at a 7–10 fold higher concentration, did not induce cytotoxicity. These results are probably due to its rapid clearance from the system. Using RBC as a vehicle for rIL2 has improved its effectiveness in generating cytotoxicity even at concentrations 6 to 8 fold less than the amount of soluble rIL2 tested. The use of RBC-rIL2 increases the serum 1/2 life of rIL2 to 3 days (DeLoach 1988); thus, providing a constant low level of IL2 as compared to a sharp peak which results from bolus IL2 injections. This constant low level of IL2 generates tumor cytotoxicity, but without the immunopathological side-effect generated by highly activated NK cells (Meir 1990).

Although IFN-γ is not detectable in the serum of mice that have been injected with RBC±rIL2, spleen cells obtained from RBC-rIL2-treated mice release much greater quantities of IFN-γ into culture upon *in vitro* LPS stimulation than those cells obtained from normal RBC-injected mice. These results indicate that IL2 exerted a priming effect on the spleen cells. It has been shown that memory cells produce much higher concentrations of IFN-γ than naive cells upon mitogenic stimulation (Sanders 1989).

Kalechman et. al. (1993) have stated that infusion of autologous RBC *in vitro* and *in vivo* resulted in an overall increase in the secretion of a number of cytokines: IL2, IFN-γ, TNF, IL6, and colony stimulating factor, plus increased IL2 receptor expression on both mouse and human cells. In our experiments, when spleen cells of tumor bearing mice (which had been injected with the various treatment groups) were cultured *in vitro*, the RBC group displayed the highest TNF and IFN-γ production. The RBC-rIL2 group also produced significantly higher amounts of IFN-γ than the soluble rIL2 and MBA injected groups. TNF and IFN-γ have both been implicated as anti-tumor cytokines (Weigent 1983, Tamura 1989, Tuttle 1992); however, increased production did not necessarily correlate with decreased tumor size in this instance. It could be postulated that the IL2 on the surface of the RBC exerts its tumoricidal activities at the beginning and as the rIL2 concentration on the RBC surface decreases, the RBC components become visible and they further stimulate the ongoing antitumor response. Most likely, in tumor bearing mice many of the activated T cells have been transported to the tumor site.

Our experiments using the RBC as a carrier for rIL2 provide promising antitumor results using very low rIL2 concentrations at weekly intervals but more importantly this paper establishes the RBC as a vehicle for expanded studies using other cytokines, antibodies, and/or drugs for tumor and disease treatment.

ACKNOWLEDGMENTS

We thank Virginia Lowry, Jan Johnson, and Ellen Moore for their technical assistance. Mention of a tradename, proprietary product, or specific equipment does not constitute a guarantee or warranty by the U.S. Department of Agriculture and does not imply its approval to the exclusion of other products that may be suitable.

6. REFERENCES

Anderson P.M., Katsanis E., Sencer S.F., Hasz D., Ochoa A.C., Bostrom B. (1992) Depot characteristics and biodistribution of interleukin-2 liposomes: importance of route of administration. *J Immunother* **12**,19–31.

Anstee D.J., Gardner B., Spring F.A., Holmes C.H., Simpson K.L., Parsons S.F., Mallinson G., Yousaf S.M., Judson P.A. (1991) New monoclonal antibodies in CD44 and CD58: their use to quantify CD44 and CD58 on normal human erythrocytes and to compare the distribution of CD44 and CD58 in human tissues. *Immunol* **74(2)**,197–205.

Cheever M.A., Thompson J.A., Kern D.E., Greenberg P.D. (1985) Interleukin-2 (IL2) administration *in vivo*: Influence of IL-2 route and timing on T cell growth. *J Immunol* **134**,3895–3900.

Cheever M.A., Thompson J.A., Peace D.J., Greenberg P.D. (1986) Potential uses of interleukin 2 in cancer therapy. *Immunobiol* **172**,365–382.

Chiarantini L., Droleskey R., Magnani M., Kirch H., DeLoach J.R. (1992) Targeting of erythrocytes to cytotoxic T cells. In *The use of resealed erythrocytes as carriers and bioreactors*. Eds. M.Magnani and J.R.DeLoach. Plenum Press, New York. p.257.

Crum E.D., Kaplan D.R. (1991) In vivo activity of solid phase interleukin 2. *Cancer Res* **51**,875–879.

DeLoach J.R., Tanger C.T., Barton C. (1983) Hepatic pharmacokinetics of glutaraldehyde treated methotrexate-loaded carrier erythrocytes in dogs. *Res Exp Med* **183**,167–175.

DeLoach J.R., Droleskey R. (1986) Survival of murine carrier erythrocytes injected via peritoneum. *Comp Biochem Physiol* **84A(3)**,447–450.

DeLoach J.R., Andrews K., Sheffield C.L. (1988) Encapsulation of interleukin-2 in murine erythrocytes and subsequent deposition in mice receiving a subcutaneous injection. *Biotech Appl Biochem* **10**,183–190.

Johnston T.P., Punjabi M.A., Froelich C.J. (1992) Sustained delivery of interleukin-2 from a poloxamer 407 gel matrix following intraperitoneal injection in mice. *Pharm Res* **9(3)**,425–434.

Kalechman Y., Herman S., Gafter U., Sredni B. (1993) Enhancing effects of autologous erythrocytes on human or mouse cytokine secretion and IL-2R expression. *Cell Immunol* **148(1)**,114–129.

Kaplan G., Cohn Z.A., Smith K.A. (1992) Rational immunotherapy with interleukin 2. *Biotech* **10**,157–162.

Lotze M.T., Chang A.E, Seipp C.A., Simpson C., Vetto J.T., Rosenberg S.A. (1986) High-dose recombinant interleukin-2 in the treatment of patients with disseminated cancer. Responses, treatment-related morbidity, and histologic findings. *JAMA* **256**,3117–3124.

Mier J.W., Vachino G., Klempner M.S., Aronson F.R., Noring R., Smith S., Brandon E.P., Laird W., Atkins M.B. (1990) Inhibition of interleukin 2 induced tumor necrosis factor release by defect and differential suppression of interleukin 2 associated side effects. *Blood* **76**,1933–1940.

Poste G., Kirsh R., Fogler W.E., Fidler I.J. (1979) Activation of tumoricidal properties in mouse macrophages by lymphokines encapsulated in liposomes. *Cancer Res* **39**,881–892.

Ritz J., Schmidt R.E., Michon J., Hercend T., Schlossman S.F. (1988) Characterization of functional surface structures on human natural killer cells. *Adv Immunol* **42**,181–211.

Ropars C., Chassaigne M., Nicolau C. (1987) *Resealed Erythrocyte as Carriers and Bioreactors*. in *Adv Biosciences* vol. 67 Pergamon Press. Oxford.

Rosenberg S.A., Lotze M.T., Muul L.M., Chang A.E., Avis F.P., Leitman S., Linehan W.M., Robertson C.N., Lee R.E., Rubin J.T., Seipp C.A., Simpson C.G., White D.E. (1987) A progress report on the treatment of 157 patients with advanced cancer using lymphokine-activated killer cells and interleukin-2 or high dose interleukin 2 alone. *N Eng J Med* **316**,889–905.

Sanders M.E., Makgoba M.W., June C.H., Young H.A., Shaw S. (1989) Enhanced responsiveness of human memory T cells to CD2 and CD3 receptor-mediated activation. *Eur J Immunol* **19(5)**,803–808.

Sosman J.A., Weiss G.R., Margolin K.A., Aronson F.R., Sznol M., Atkins M.B., O'Boyle K., Fisher S.G., Mier J., Vachino G., Caliendo G. (1993) Phase I B clinical trial of anti-CD3 followed by high-dose bolus interleukin-2 in patients with metastatic melanoma and advanced renal cell carcinoma: clinical and immunological effects. *J Clin Oncol* **11**,1496–1505.

Tamura K., Aso H., Nakamura T., Hemmi H., Ishida N. (1989) Evaluation of recombinant human tumor necrosis factor by scheduled intratumoral administration in mice bearing transplatable tumor. *Tohoku J. Exp. Med*, **157**,107–118.

Thrombe P.S., Deodhar S.D. (1984) Inhibition of liver metastases in murine colon adenocarcinoma by liposomes containing human c-reactive protein or crude lymphokine. *Cancer Immunol Immunother* **16**,145–150.

Tuttle T.M., McCrady C.W., Inge T.H., Salour M., Bear H.D. (1992) γ–Interferon plays a key role in T cell induced tumor regression. *Cancer Research* **53**,833–839.

Weigent D.A., Stanton G.J., Johnson H.M. (1983) Interleukin 2 enhances natural killer cell activity through induction of gamma interferon. *Infect Imm* **41**,992–997.32.

2

HUMAN RECOMBINANT INTERLEUKIN 2 BINDS TO MOUSE RED BLOOD CELLS VIA THE ERYTHROPOIETIN RECEPTOR

Rita B. Moyes and John R. DeLoach

USDA-ARS-FAPRL
Collcgc Station, Tcxas 77845

1. ABSTRACT

Murine red blood cells (RBC) incubated with recombinant human interleukin 2 (rIL2) bound 10–20% of the added cytokine with 41.28 ± 4.64% of the population positive for bound cytokine as determined by fluorescence activated cell scanning (FACS) analysis. It has been well documented that a high degree of homology exists between the erythropoietin receptor (EPOR) and the IL2βR chain (based both on amino acid sequence and hydrophobicity alignment), we hypothesized that the rIL2 was binding to residual EPOR on murine RBC. Upon bioassay, it was found that reticulocytes (RET), which express a higher percentage of EPOR than normal RBC, bound 400% more rIL2 as compared to normal RBC. FACS analysis using fluorescently labeled rIL2 revealed a log higher fluorescence intensity on RET compared to RBC. Therefore, the population of immature or young RBC in circulation which are expressing residual EPOR are binding rIL2 due to cross-reactivity between the EPOR and IL2βR.

2. INTRODUCTION

Interleukin 2 (IL2), a lymphocytotrophic hormone secreted exclusively by stimulated T cells (Smith 1984), is a principle regulator of both humoral and cell mediated immunity and stimulates a variety of cell types by interacting with its specific cell surface receptor. The interleukin 2 receptor (IL2R) consists of various combinations of the alpha, beta, and gamma chains which regulate the affinity of the receptor (Waldman 1993). Some of the cells that have been identified which express various chains of the IL2R include T cells, B cells, large granular lymphocytes (Waldman 1993), neutrophils (Djeu 1993), monocytes (Kniep 1992), NK cells (Nagler 1990), mast cells, and basophils (Maggiano 1990).

Erythrocytes as Drug Carriers in Medicine, edited by Sprandel and Way
Plenum Press, New York, 1997

The IL2R has not been previously demonstrated on the red blood cell (RBC) although several other immunologically relevant receptors have been identified including a chemokine receptor (Horuk 1993), which binds IL8, a prostaglandin E1 receptor (Dutta-Roy 1993), complement receptor type 1 (Paccaud 1988), as well as CD58 (Kalechman 1993) and CD44 (Anstee 1991) adhesion molecules. Additionally, RBC augment natural killer cell cytotoxicity by a natural killer enhancing factor found in the RBC's cytosol (Shau 1993). The RBC is not the inert oxygen carrier as once supposed but does show some potential for immunoregulatory functions based on the presence of these immunological receptors.

In previous studies, it has been shown that rIL2 readily adsorbs onto the RBC surface in protein free media without losing its bioactivity (DeLoach 1991). Approximately 20% of the added cytokine bound to the RBC (Kirch 1994). When rIL2-coated RBC (RBC-IL2) were incubated in protein containing media for 24 hr, washed, then transferred to fresh media containing an IL2-dependent cytotoxic T cell line (CTLL), the RBC-IL2 were able to supply IL2 for CTLL proliferation (Kirch 1994). Recombinant IL2 on the RBC surface displays extensive self-association and aggregation (Fleishmann 1988); thus, rIL2 becomes available in soluble form for cellular interaction. However, experimental evidence demonstrates that surface bound IL2 is also biologically active (DeLoach 1991).

Originally, we believed that the rIL2 binding to the RBC was a nonspecific interaction. However, D'Andrea and colleagues cloned the erythropoietin receptor (EPOR), which upon examination, revealed extensive homology to the IL2βR chain (D'Andrea 1990). The EPOR and IL2βR chain can be aligned based on regions of hydrophobicity and amino acid sequence identity. Additionally, the two receptors share several structural features: both are 500 amino acid type 1 membrane-spanning proteins (D'Andrea 1990) and have been placed in a new family of receptors based on a set of 4 conserved cysteine residues and a 5 residue motif (Trp-Ser-X-Trp-Ser) located near the transmembrane domain (D'Andra 1989). We hypothesized that due to the similarity in structure the rIL2 was binding to residual EPOR on the mouse RBC. Since cells beyond the erythroblast stage of development are no longer dependent on EPO, the number of receptors per cell is greatly reduced (Koury 1988). Thus, the RET, being a developmentally more immature cell than the RBC, should bind more rIL2. In this study, we used various techniques to test this hypothesis by measuring differences in rIL2 binding to RET and RBC.

3. MATERIALS AND METHODS

3.1. Media and Buffer

RPMI 1640 (Sigma, St. Louis,MO) was supplemented with 2mM L-glutamine (Sigma), and 5% antibiotic/antimycotic solution (Sigma) in all cases, and with 5% fetal bovine serum (FBS) (Sigma) for cell culture (RPMI-FBS). RBC and RET were washed in a PBS buffer containing 10mM glucose, 4mM $MgCl_2$, 5 mM adenosine, and 5 mM inosine (Sigma) referred to as mouse buffer A (MBA).

3.2. Antibodies

The antibodies (Ab) used in this study include: sheep polyclonal anti-human erythropoietin (EPO) receptor Ab (Upstate Biotechnology, Lake Placid, NY), rat anti-mouse IL2βR-fluorescein isothiocyanate (FITC) labeled Ab (Pharmingen, San Diego,

CA), rat anti-mouse IL2αR-pycoerythrin (PE) labeled Ab (Boehringer Mannheim, Indianapolis, IN), goat anti-rabbit IgG-FITC labeled Ab and donkey anti-sheep IgG-FITC labeled Ab (Sigma).

3.3. Cell Line

An IL2 dependent cytotoxic T cell line, CTLL (TIB 214, ATCC,Rockville, MD) was maintained on RPMI-FBS with the addition of T-stim (Collaborative Biomedical Products, Bedford, MA), an IL2 supplement.

3.4. Mice

Female Balb/c mice were purchased from Harlan Laboratories (Houston, TX). The mice were housed and fed ad libitum according to the USDA guidelines established by the Animal Care and Use Committee.

3.5. Cytokine

Recombinant human IL2 was purchased from Cellular Products (Buffalo, NY). Each vial contained 100ug/ml of rIL2 (15.4kD) and was stabilized in a 2% FBS solution. Recombinant human IL2 differs from natural IL2 in that it is not glycosylated and differs at two amino acid positions (the first 3 N-terminal amino acids are absent and cys at position 125 is substituted by ser). Recombinant hIL2-PE labeled for use in cell surface labeling experiments was purchased from R&D Systems (Minneapolis, MN).

3.6. Isolation of Erythrocytes

Mice were euthanized with CO_2 and blood was collected via cardiac puncture. The RBC were washed 3 times with MBA at 400 x g at 4°C for 10 minutes. The buffy coat was removed and discarded after the first wash. Erythrocytes were counted using a computerized Coulter counter (Hileah, FL) and were resuspended in MBA to a concentration of 10^{10}cells per ml. Blood smear analysis demonstrated RBC with <1% RET and <1% leukocytes (WBC).

3.7. Production of Reticulocytes

Mice were made anemic by i.p. injection of 200ul of a 0.075% solution of phenylhydrazine (Sigma) in MBA for 3 consecutive days followed by 3 to 5 days of rest. The cells were then collected as described above in isolation of erythrocytes. Blood smear analysis revealed approximately 50% RET.

3.8. Binding of rIL2

RBC and RET were resuspended in separate sterile eppendorf tubes (USA Scientific, Ocala, FL) to 10^{10} cells per ml and incubated with rIL2 at a ratio of 400ul rIL2/10^{10} cells (1.44 x 10^6 IU/ml of rIL2) with gentle rotation for 30 min at 4°C. The cells were then washed 3 times with 4 volumes of MBA. This technique yielded approximately 10,000–12,000 IU of rIL2 coated on the surface per 10^9 erythrocytes as determined by the

CTLL bioassay described below. Normal RBC were prepared by incubation in the same volume MBA for 30 minutes at 4°C followed by 3 washes.

3.9. Bioassay of Erythrocyte-Bound rIL2

RBC-rIL2 and RET-rIL2 at 10^{10} cells/ml were carried through 3 freeze/thaw cycles to assure complete lysis of the cell. Dilutions in complete media were made and 50ul of each dilution were added to 200ul of CTLL cells (10^6 cells/ml) in a 96 well flat bottom plate. The plates were incubated for 20 hours at 37°C in 5% CO_2 and then pulsed with 0.4 uCi/well of [3H]thymidine (ICN, Irvine, CA) for the final 4 hours. Cells were harvested using a Skatron cell harvester (Sterling, VA) onto glass fiber filters and [3H] thymidine incorporation was determined by liquid scintillation counting. Normal RBC were lysed and used as control supernatants and rIL2 standards were used to construct calibration curves for assessing levels of IL2 bound to the RBC and RET surface.

3.10. FACS Analysis

One hundred microliters of MBA +1% BSA containing 1 x 10^6 cells was added to each eppendorf tube and the primary antibody was added as indicated by the manufacturer. If the primary antibody was not labeled then a secondary fluorescently labeled anti-

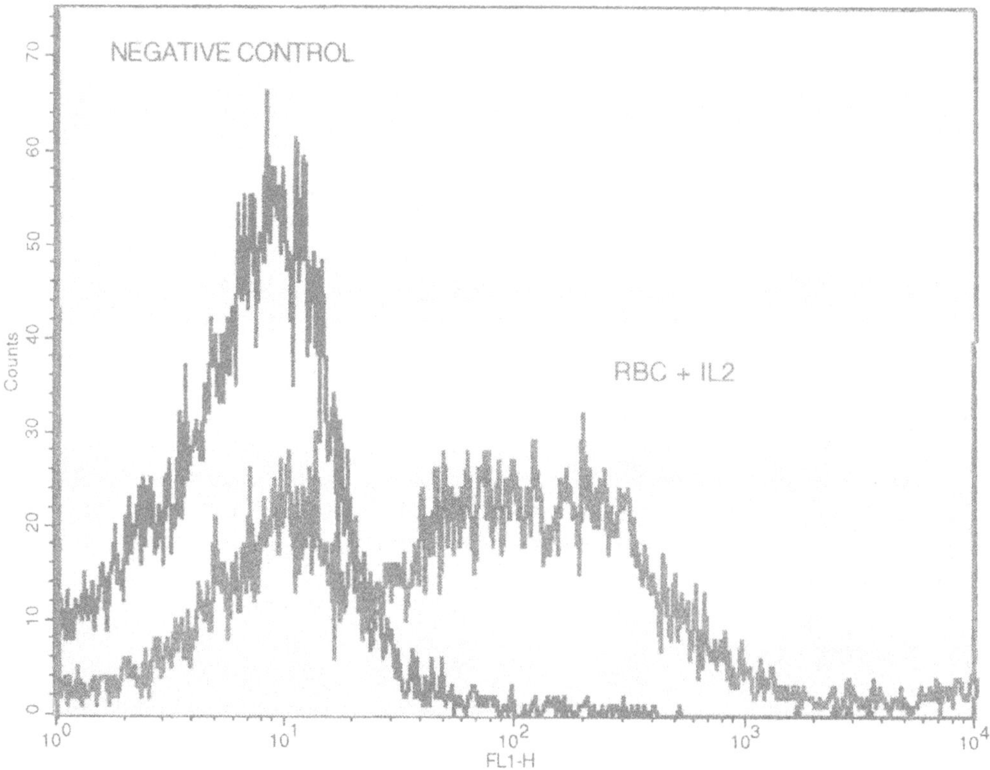

Figure 1. Representative FACS profile of RBC labeled with IL2 as visualized by IL2 + anti-IL2 + anti-rabbit IgG-FITC Ab. The negative control is RBC + anti-rabbit IgG-FITC.

body was introduced after the first incubation. All incubations took place at 4°C for 1 hr with gentle agitation and each incubation was followed by 3 washes in MBA+1% BSA. When cells were labeled with rIL2 or EPO, cells were incubated with 20ul of rIL2 or 4 ul of EPO for 30 minutes at 4°C with rocking, washed, then the primary antibody was introduced. After staining, all cells were fixed in 500 ul of a 1.5% paraformaldehyde solution in MBA. Cells were also labeled with irrelevant isotype-matched labeled antibodies to serve as non-specific antibody binding controls. Fluorescence intensity of 10^4 cells per sample was analyzed by quantitative flow cytometry using a FACSCAN (Becton Dickinson, San Jose, CA).

4. RESULTS

4.1. Binding of rIL2 and Antibody to Cells

Recombinant human IL2 binds to 41.3± 4.6% of murine RBC when incubated at 4°C for 30 minutes in protein-free media (Figure 1). An IL2 dependent cell line, CTLL, was used as a control for all of the IL2 experiments and is 79% positive for IL2 binding (Table 1). In both cell types, RBC and CTLL cells, the percentage of IL2 positive cells is essentially the same as that seen with anti-IL2βR binding (Table 1). This result is expected for CTLL cells since they express a definitive IL2R to which the IL2 is binding. However, IL2-IL2βR binding has not been previously described for the RBC. The anti-IL2βR Ab

Table 1. FACS analysis of IL2, anti-IL2R, and anti-EPOR binding to RBC as compared to CTLL cells, an IL2-dependent line, and competition of binding

	percent positive cells	
treatment	CTLL	RBC
1. IL2+α-IL2+α-Rab IgG-FITC	79.74±2.51 (7)*b	41.28±4.64 (9)B,‡
2. α-IL2βR-FITC	81.07±14.61 (3)	31.67±6.25 (6)B, †
3. α-IL2αR-PE	11.53±3.84 (3)a,b,c	1.40±0.63 (4)A,B,C,†
4. IL2+α-IL2βR-FITC	75.67±12.98 (3)	43.0±0.71 (3)B
5. α-EPOR+α-Sheep IgG-FITC	58.58±9.69 (4)a	91.93±3.18 (8)A,C,‡
6. α-EPOR+IL2+α-IL2+α-Rab IgG-FITC	66.99±5.57 (7)a	51.97±5.59 (6)B
7. IL2+α-EPOR+α-Sheep IgG-FITC	65.88±7.43 (6)a	95.60±4.47 (3)A,C,†
8. EPO+IL2+α-IL2+α-RAB IgG-FITC	51.40±0.20 (3)a	N.D.
9. EPO+α-EPOR+α-Sheep IgG-FITC	39.74±0.20 (3)a	2.42±2.64 (3)A,B,C,‡

*(n)= number of experimental replicates. All values represent the percentage obtained when the negatives were gated to <5% positive. The negative controls for this experiment consisted of cells reacted with the anti-rabbit and anti-sheep-FITC labeled secondary antibodies to compensate for nonspecific antibody binding.

The student's t test was performed using the MicroCal Origin Software Package (Northampton, MA) to compare the data as indicated.

Within the CTLL group:

a=data compared to IL2 binding (treatment group 1) $p<0.05$

b=data compared to anti-EPOR Ab binding (treatment group 5) $p<0.05$

c=data compared to anti-IL2βR Ab binding (treatment group 2) $p<0.01$

Within the RBC group:

A= data compared to IL2 binding $p<0.001$

B=data compared to anti-EPOR Ab binding $p<0.0001$

C=data compared to anti-IL2βR Ab binding $p<0.05$

Between CTLL and RBC results:

†$p<0.05$

‡$p<0.001$

used in these studies is not a blocking Ab for IL2 binding and prior binding of IL2 does not block the binding of the Ab to the surface of the cells (Table 1). Even though a small percentage (11.5%) of IL2αR can be detected on the CTLL cells, the RBC are negative for this IL2 receptor (1.4%, Table 1).

An anti-murine EPOR Ab was not available for our research purposes; however, since there is 82% homology (Youssofian 1993) between human and mouse EPOR, we decided to test anti-human EPOR Ab in our system. When tested with anti-human EPOR Ab, both RBC and CTLL cells (92 and 59% positive, respectively) which are of mouse origin labeled significantly with the anti-EPOR Ab (Table 1). There is no statistical difference of binding on the CTLL cells by anti-IL2βR and anti-EPOR Ab due to the large standard deviation. Thus, the two Ab are recognizing the same receptor on the cell surface just different epitopes on that receptor. The binding of the anti-EPOR Ab can be completely blocked by prior incubation of the RBC with rEPO; however, the Ab was not affected by prior IL2 binding (Figure 2). Likewise, the binding of anti-EPOR Ab to CTLL cells was not blocked by prior binding of IL2 but it was partially blocked by EPO binding (Table 1). Therefore, EPO and IL2 are not binding to the same epitope expressed by the cell surface receptor; however, EPO is binding to or blocking the epitope recognized by the anti-EPOR Ab on RBC. Due to the partial blocking of IL2 binding to the CTLL cells

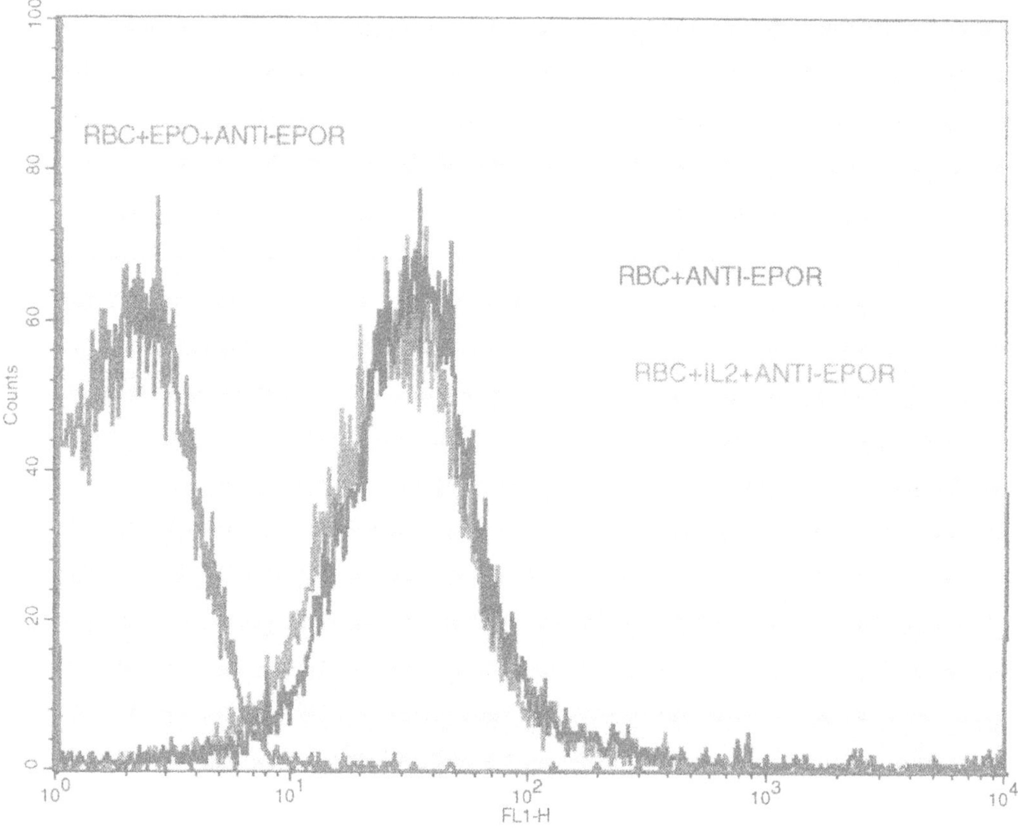

Figure 2. Flow cytometric analysis of RBC reacted with anti-human EPOR Ab which was labeled with anti-sheep IgG-FITC Ab. RBC were also pre-incubated with EPO and IL2 before anti-EPOR Ab binding in order to evaluate any blocking effects for subsequent Ab binding by these compounds.

by EPO and anti-EPOR, the binding of EPO and anti-EPOR must be sterically hindering the binding of IL2 is some instances.

4.2. Comparison of Cell Bound rIL2 on Reticulocytes versus Erythrocytes

Bioassay of RBC-IL2 confirmed the presence of IL2 on the RBC which was biologically capable of supporting the IL2 dependent CTLL cell line (Table 2). Compared to the media control, sham treated RBC and RET (no IL2) also did not support cellular proliferation. From the bioassay, it appears that the RET-IL2 are carrying larger quantities of IL2 on their surface than RBC-IL2 as evidenced by the increased proliferation (Table 2). When actual bound IL2 concentrations were calculated from known IL2 standards, the RET bound 4.3 ± 0.73 times as much IL2 on their cell surface as did normal RBC ($p<.001$, Table 3).

Analysis of IL2 binding on the cell surface of RET versus RBC was accomplished using fluorescently labeled IL2 (IL2-PE) Figure 3. The RBC population yielded one peak shifted slightly to the right of the negative control (cells incubated with PE labeled streptavidin). However, RET demonstrated a bimodal population with the first peak overlapping the RBC peak and the second peak displaying a log higher fluorescence which translates to increased IL2-PE binding per cell. Our procedure for RET enrichment yields a 40–60% RET population. Therefore, the RET, with higher EPOR numbers, constitute the more intense peak with the normal RBC within the population mirroring the whole RBC population. It is interesting to note that even a portion of the RBC population peak is positive compared to the negative control, just less IL2 is bound per cell. This supports the theory that the EPOR must persist in some form to various degrees on the mature RBC.

5. DISCUSSION

Initial encapsulation experiments using recombinant human IL2 revealed that a certain amount of the cytokine was retained on the cell surface despite repeated washings. Both the pellet and lysate of the RBC with encapsulated rIL2 were able to sustain the growth of CTLL cells (DeLoach 1991). These findings have been corroborated with mouse, sheep, and human cells using various rIL2 formulations (DeLoach 1988,1991).

Table 2. Representative results of CTLL proliferation whe tested with cell-bound rIL2

test lysate	CTLL proliferation (dpm)
media only	9186
normal RBC	8959
normal RET	9520
RBC-IL2	126,511
RET-IL2	286,268

fifty microliters of freeze/thaw lysate of 10^{10} cells/ml were subjected to non-serial dilutions and tested in the CTLL assay. The counts of the IL2 coated cells are from the 1:2000 dilution in order for the counts to fall within the range of the rIL2 standard curve.

Table 3. Comparison of bound human rIL2 on murine reticulocytes versus erythrocytes as determined by CTLL bioassay

	RET		RBC
rIL2 IU/10^9 cells	149,108 ±32,203		38,378 ±5984
RET:RBC [rIL2]		3.9±0.73*	

n= 8 experiments with each experiment the average of three sample determinations per cell type.

*The ratio of the mean IL2 concentration bound to RET as compared to RBC was significantly greater ($p<.001$) using a one-tailed ANOVA test.

Preliminary experiments in our laboratory (Moyes 1994) using RBC-IL2 as a therapeutic delivery system in the mouse demonstrated the presence of anti-IL2 Ab, increased tumor cytotoxicity, and increased interferon gamma production. All of these parameters indicate that the IL2 was biologically active after being bound to the RBC. Due to the therapeutic potential of the RBC-IL2 system, we wanted to determine the nature of the IL2 binding. Studies using anti-IL2 Ab followed by a secondary FITC-labeled Ab revealed that about 40% of the RBC population from normal mice were capable of binding a detectable amount of rIL2 on their surface. FACS analysis revealed a dual peak, one that was in-

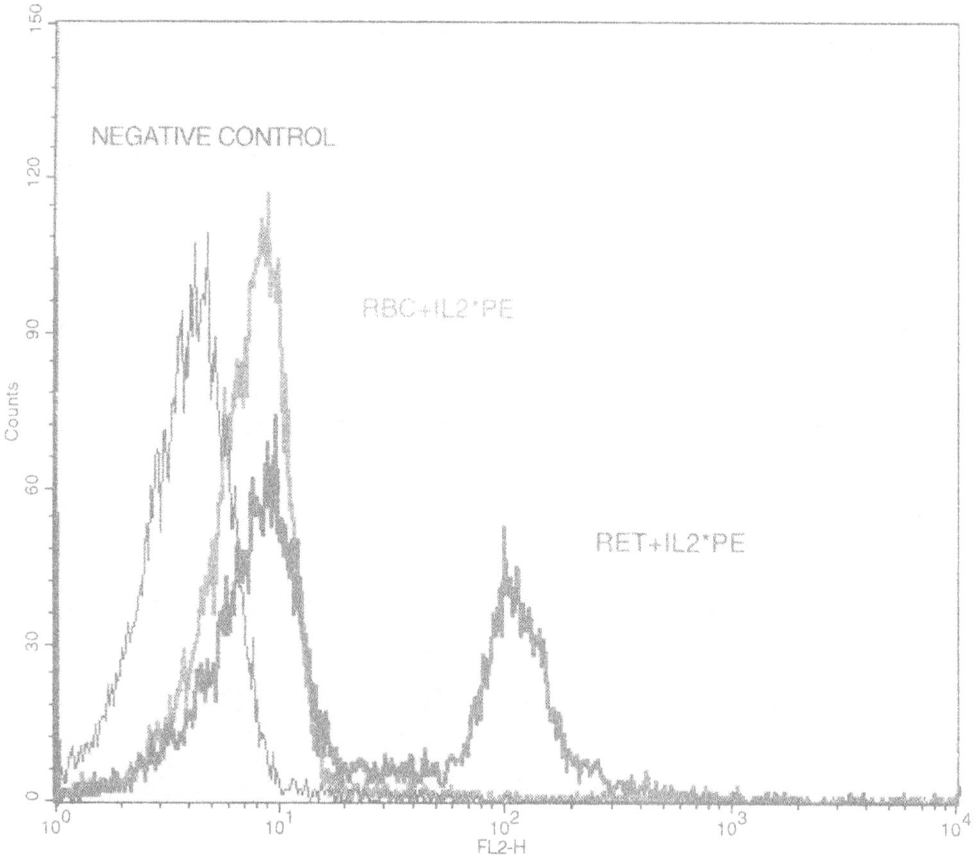

Figure 3. Flow cytometric comparison of PE-labeled IL2 binding to normal murine RBC versus an enriched RET population. The negative control consisted of RBC and RET reacted with PE-labeled streptavidin. The RBC control is pictured in the figure as a representative negative control for both cell types.

tensely fluorescent and a peak that corresponded to the negative control. This finding led us to believe that a certain RBC subpopulation was expressing some type of receptor or protein that allowed the IL2 to bind. If rIL2 is added to erythrocytes in the presence of plasma, all of the rIL2 remains in the soluble fraction (DeLoach 1988). Therefore, extraneous proteins must coat the RBC surface and subsequently inhibit rIL2 binding. This reasoning explains why natural IL2 does not bind to the RBC *in vivo*. Our washing probably strips "protective" proteins from the RBC surface thus revealing cryptic receptors such as a low-affinity or partial EPOR which become available for rIL2 binding *in vitro*. Research by D'Andrea et al. (D'Andrea 1989, 1990) outlined the similarities and sequence homologies shared between the IL2βR and EPOR both at the amino acid sequence level and regional hydrophobicity level. Like the IL2R, the EPOR also exists in more than one state of affinity which has led many to believe that the high affinity EPOR is due to a 2-chain heterodimeric receptor (D'Andrea 1990) and that EPO-unresponsive cell lines, e.g. murine erythroleukemia cells only express the low-affinity receptor. Landschulz et al. (1989) examined the EPO binding and response in murine erythroid progenitor cells and found that the EPOR undergoes rapid turnover with high-affinity receptors disappearing 7–8 hours into culture but the low-affinity receptors were undiminished at up to 16 hrs. The authors stated that at least 2 gene products regulated EPO binding with the high-affinity receptors mediating the maturation effects of EPO during the first 8 hrs of culture. They further hypothesized that the persistent low-affinity receptors must be involved in some yet to be defined function of EPO. Therefore, there is evidence of persistence of low-affinity EPOR on the erythroid surface.

It is known that as RBC age, their surface undergoes changes with some receptors disappearing and new or cryptic proteins being uncovered as the surface changes. Unlike other cell types, RBC lack surface protein turnover to any appreciable extent. The RBC surface is modified instead by covalent aggregation, nonenzymatic glycosylation, proteolytic degradation, and carboxyl methylation (Bartosz 1991). Each of these biochemical modifications could play a part in altering the functional and antigenic sites of a low affinity EPOR. Our repeated washings may have removed some blocking or cross-linked proteins making the EPOR again available for Ab recognition. The anti-human EPOR Ab reacted with a much higher percentage of the RBC population than was expected. However, this result may be a fortuitous discovery in that the anti-human Ab recognizes a cryptic site on the murine receptor that normally would not induce an Ab response when the murine EPOR was used as an immunogen. The fact that Ab isotype matched controls do not demonstrate nonspecific binding to the RBC surface and that prior EPO binding totally blocks the Ab interaction points to a true EPOR epitope. When flow cytometry studies were done with EPO followed by anti-EPO, no binding of the anti-EPO could be detected. The altered state of the EPOR may have allowed binding of EPO but in a less conventional way. This altered EPO binding was able to block anti-EPOR binding but had somehow hidden the binding site on EPO from its anti-EPO Ab.

The fact that IL2-PE binding to a RET enriched population demonstrated 2 peaks leads to several conclusions. Both populations were positive for IL2 binding although the RET population demonstrated more binding sites per cell as evidenced by increased fluorescent intensity. Therefore, a receptor was still available for IL2 binding on the normal RBC population. At this point it should be stressed that the entire peak representing the RET population was positive for IL2 binding while the normal RBC peak was approximately 45% positive for IL2 binding as compared to the negative control. We postulate that there is a continuing but gradual loss or degradation of the receptor as the RBC ages. Future experiments using isolated aged RBC with subsequent IL2-PE binding will verify this assumption. These results correspond with our initial labeling experiments in which IL2, labeled with an anti-IL2 Ab followed by a secondary FITC-labeled Ab, yielded about 40% of the RBC labeled with IL2 (Figure 1, Table 1). Reticulocyte stain analysis of our normal RBC populations produced <1% of the cells classified as RET, so that suggests that mature RBC were being labeled. Preliminary RT-PCR experiments have demonstrated no detectable IL2βR mRNA from mouse RET as compared to positive CTLL cell controls (data not shown). In addition, D'Andrea et al. (1990) have already determined the absence of IL2αR mRNA from erythroid lines when looking for an IL2R tac-like subunit for the EPOR. Therefore, we do not believe that a definitive IL2βR exists on the RBC.

In conclusion, we hypothesize from our experimental evidence that human rIL2 and anti-IL2βR Ab are binding to the RBC in a cross-reactive manner with the EPOR due to its similarity in structure to the IL2βR, and that this phenomenon is not seen *in vivo* with natural IL2 because of interfering proteins on the RBC and its milieu.

ACKNOWLEDGMENTS

The authors thank Virginia Lowry for her expert technical assistance. Mention of a tradename, proprietary product, or specific equipment does not constitute a guarantee or warranty by the U.S. Department of Agriculture and does not imply its approval to the exclusion of other products that may be suitable.

6. REFERENCES

Anstee, N.J., Gardner, B.K., Spring, F.A., Holmes, C.H., Simpson, K.L., Parsons, S.F., Mallinson, G., Yousaf, S.M., Judson, P.A.New monoclonal antibodies in CD44 and CD58:their use to quantify CD44 and CD58 on normal human erythrocytes and to compare the distribution of CD44 and CD58 in human tissues. Immunol. 74, 197–205, 1991.

Bartosz, G. Erythrocyte aging: physical and chemical membrane changes. Gerontology 37, 33–67, 1991.

D'Andrea, A.D., Fasman, G., Wong, G., Lodish, H. Erythropoietin receptor: cloning strategy and structural features. Intl. J. of Cell Cloning 8(suppl 1), 173–180, 1990.

D'Andrea, A.D., Fasman, G.D., Lodish, H. Erythropoietin receptor and interleukin-2 receptor β chain: a new receptor family. Cell 58, 1023–1024, 1989.

DeLoach, J.R., Andrews, K., Kruse, C. Encapsulation of human recombinant interleukin-2 into carrier erythrocytes by hypoosmotic dialysis and its subsequent biological activity. Adv. Biosciences 81, 59–65, 1991.

DeLoach, J.R., Andrews, K., Sheffield, C.L. Encapsulation of Interleukin-2 in murine erythrocytes and subsequent deposition in mice receiving a subcutaneous injection. Biotech. Appl. Biochem. 10, 183–190, 1988.

Djeu, J.Y., Liu, J.H., Wei, S., Rui,H., Pearson, C.A., Leonard, W.J., Blanchard, D.K. Function associated with IL2 receptor β on human neutrophils: mechanism of activation of antifungal activity against *Candida albicans* by IL2. J. Immunol. 150, 960–970, 1993.

Dutta-Roy, A.K., Hoque, L., Paterson, B.J. Prostaglandin-E1-binding sites in rabbit erythrocyte membranes. Eur. J. Biochem. 213, 1167–1173, 1993.

Fleishmann, J.D., Wentworth, D., Valencic, F., Imbembo, A.L., Kochler, K.A. Interleukin 2 self-association. Biochem. Biophys. Res. Comm. 152(2), 879–885, 1988.

Horuk, R., Colby, T.J., Darbonne, W.C., Schall, T.J., Neote, K.The human erythrocyte inflammatory peptide (chemokine) receptor. Biochemical charaterization, solubilization, and development of a binding assay for the soluble receptor. Biochem. 32, 5733–5738, 1993.

Kalechman, Y., Herman, S., Gafter, U., and Sredni, B. Enhancing effects of autologous erythrocytes on human or mouse cytokine secretion and IL-2R expression. Cell. Immunol. 148, 114–129, 1993.

Kirch, H.J., Moyes, R.B., Chiarantini, L., DeLoach, J.R. Effect of targeted erythrocytes coated with recombinant human interleukin 2 on T-lymphocyte proliferation *in vitro*. Biotechnol. Appl. Biochem. 19, 331–340, 1994.

Kniep, E.M., Strelow, I., Lohman-Matthes, M.-L. The monocyte interleukin-2 receptor light chain: production of cell-associated and soluble interleukin-2 receptor by monocytes. Immunol. 75, 299–304, 1992.

Koury, M.J., Bondurant, M.C. Maintenance by erythropoietin of viability and maturation of murine erythroid precursor cells. J. Cell. Physiol. 137, 65–74, 1988.

Landschulz, K.T., Noyes, A.N., Rogers, O., Boyer, S.H. Erythropoeitin receptors on murine erythroid colony-forming units: natural history. Blood 73, 1476–1486, 1989.

Maggiano, N., Colotta, F., Castellino, F., Ricci, R.,Valitutti, S., Larocca, L.M., Musiani, P.Interleukin-2 receptor expression in human mast cells and basophils. Int. Arch. Allergy Appl. Immunol. 91, 8–14, 1990.

Moyes, R.B., Kirch, H.J., DeLoach, J.R. Immunotherapeutic evaluation of human recombinant interleukin 2 (rIL2) coated erythrocytes using the murine model. Adv Biosciences 92, 151–162, 1993.

Nagler, A., Lanier, L.L., Phillips, J.H. Constitutive expression of high affinity interleukin 2 receptors on human CD16-natural killer cells *in vivo*. J. Exp. Med. 171, 1527–1533, 1990

Paccaud, J.P., Carpentier, J.L., Schifferli, J.A.Direct evidence for the clustered nature of complement receptors type I on the erythrocyte membrane. J. Immunol. 141, 3889–3894, 1988.

Shau, H., Gupta, R.K., Golub, S.H. Identification of a natural killer enhancing factor (NKEF) from human erythroid cells. Cell. Immunol. 147, 1–11, 1993.

Smith,K.A. Interleukin 2. Ann. Rev. Immunol. 2, 319–333,1984.

Waldman, T.A.The IL-2/IL-2 receptor system: a target for rational immune intervention. Imm. Today 14, 264–270, 1993.

Youssofian, H., Longmore, G., Neumann, D., Yoshimura, A., Lodish, H. Structure, function, and activation of the erythropoietin receptor. Blood 81(9), 2223–2236, 1993.

3

IN VIVO SURVIVAL OF HUMAN ENERGY-REPLETE CARRIER ERYTHROCYTES

Murray D. Bain,[1] Bridget E. Bax,[1] Peter J. Talbot,[2] E. John Parker-Williams,[2] and Ronald A. Chalmers[1]

[1]Paediatric Metabolism Unit
Department of Child Health
[2]Department of Haematology
St. George's Hospital Medical School
London, United Kingdom

1. INTRODUCTION

Erythrocytes have been proposed as carriers of encapsulated therapeutic agents. Encapsulation of therapeutic agents within erythrocytes with a normal mean cell life range of 89 to 131 days (normal half-life of 19 to 29 days) should limit the vascular clearance of the administered drug thus reducing the dosage and frequency of therapeutic interventions.

We have recently demonstrated that therapeutic enzyme entrapment can be increased by extending the hypo-osmotic dialysis time of human carrier erythrocytes (Bax et al., 1996a; 1996b). However to be successful as a sustained therapeutic agent delivery system it is essential to first demonstrate that carrier erythrocytes have a near physiological survival time *in vivo*. We have previously reported in preliminary form the *in vivo* survival of human carrier erythrocytes (Bax et al., 1996c). We now report the *in vivo* survival of unloaded carrier erythrocytes prepared using the two different hypo-osmotic dialysis times that we employed in our *in vitro* entrapment studies.

2. MATERIALS AND METHODS

2.1. Volunteers

Nine healthy volunteers (4 females and 5 males) aged 21 to 43 years (mean 25.6) were used in this study. Ethical approval was granted by the Local Research Ethics Committee.

Erythrocytes as Drug Carriers in Medicine, edited by Sprandel and Way
Plenum Press, New York, 1997

2.2. Blood Preparation

Sterile materials and aseptic conditions were used throughout. Forty ml of blood were collected and placed into 2 tubes containing 4 ml anticoagulant citrate dextrose BP (n=2) or 200 units heparin BP (n=7). The blood samples were centrifuged for 10 minutes at 1100g; the supernatant plasma was removed and kept for later use and the buffy coat was discarded. The erythrocytes were washed twice in cold (4°C) phosphate buffered saline (PBS), pH 7.4 (2.68 mmol/l KCl, 1.47 mmol/l KH_2PO_4, 136.89 mmol/l NaCl, 8.10 mmol/l Na_2HPO_4) and centrifuged for 10 minutes at 1100g.

2.3. Carrier Erythrocyte Preparation

Energy-replete carrier erythrocytes were prepared using a hypo-osmotic dialysis technique (Sprandel, Hubbard and Chalmers, 1980; 1981). Washed and packed fresh erythrocytes (10.5 ml) were mixed with cold PBS to a final haematocrit of 70%. Five ml of cell suspension were placed into each of three dialysis bags (molecular weight cut-off of 12,000 daltons, Medicell International Ltd, London) which were then sealed at both ends with clips. Each dialysis bag was placed into a container and supported firmly by wedging the dialysis clips against the container side. Dialysis was against 150 ml hypo-osmotic phosphate buffer, pH 7.4 (5 mmol/l KH_2PO_4, 5 mmol/l K_2HPO_4) at 4°C in a Lab-Heat refrigerated incubator (Boro Labs Ltd, Berkshire) for 90 (n=6) or 180 (n=3) minutes, with rotation at 6 rpm. The lysed erythrocytes were resealed by transferring the dialysis bags to containers holding 150 ml PBS supplemented with 5 mmol/l adenosine, 5 mmol/l glucose and 5 mmol/l $MgCl_2$ (supplemented PBS), and continuing rotation at 6 rpm in the incubator, now at 37°C, for 60 minutes. The energy-replete carrier erythrocytes were washed three times in 3 volumes supplemented PBS with centrifugation at 100g for 15 minutes and finally pooled.

2.4. Labelling of Carrier Erythrocytes with Sodium [^{51}Cr] Chromate

Carrier erythrocytes were labelled using a standard ^{51}Cr erythrocyte-labelling technique (International Committee for Standardization in Haematology, 1980); the washed and packed cells were gently mixed with 0.75 MBq Sodium [^{51}Cr] chromate BP (Amersham International, Buckinghamshire) and allowed to stand at room temperature for 30 minutes. Unbound chromium was removed with either 100 mg ascorbic acid BP (100 mg/ml, Evans Medical, Leatherhead) which reduces the chromate ion to the non-permeable chromic followed by a single wash in supplemented PBS (n=7) or by 3 washes in supplemented PBS (n=2). Following resuspension in an equal volume of autologous plasma, the carrier erythrocytes were injected slowly over a period of 5 minutes into the volunteer's arm vein.

2.5. Assessment of Carrier Erythrocyte Survival

In vivo survival was assessed by monitoring the disappearance of label from the circulation; 10 ml blood samples were taken from a vein in the opposing arm 15, 30, 60, 120 and 180 minutes after injection, then twice in the first week and weekly until activity was not noticeably above background. To check for intra vascular haemolysis, plasma was measured for ^{51}Cr activity. Urinary excretion of label was assessed in 7 volunteers by making 24 hour urine collections for the first 72 hours after injection. ^{51}Cr activity in the liver, spleen and heart was measured up to 144 hours after injection by surface counting using a gamma counter (John Caunt Scientific, Oxfordshire) in 7 volunteers; the liver and spleen were surface counted because these are sites of erythrocyte sequestration and destruction and surface counting the heart gives a measure of circulating labelled cells.

3. RESULTS

3.1. Cell Survival

Between 3 and 24 hours after injection 55.5% (mean of the lowest activities recorded during this period, 90 minutes of hypo-osmotic dialysis) and 49.1% (mean, 180 minutes of hypo-osmotic dialysis) of the injected labelled carrier erythrocytes had disappeared from the circulation. The label in the circulation then increased between 24 and 96 hours by 27.8% (mean; the individual values calculated from the difference between the lowest recorded levels between 3 and 24 hours and the highest recorded levels between 24 and 96 hours, and expressed as a percentage of the lowest value) for 90 minutes of hypo-osmotic dialysis and 8.5% (mean) for 180 minutes hypo-osmotic dialysis (Figure 1).

Unloaded carrier erythrocytes prepared using both 90 minutes and 180 minutes of hypo-osmotic dialysis had *in vivo* mean cell half-lives and mean cell survivals within the normal range; the mean cell half-life was 27 ± 3.6 (mean ± SD of 6 subjects) and 29 ± 5.3 days (mean ± SD of 3 subjects) for 90 and 180 minutes of hypo-osmotic dialysis respectively, well within the normal range of 19 to 29 days. There were no significant differences between the two hypo-osmotic dialysis times, $p>0.5$ (Table 1).

The mean cell life (MCL) was 106 ± 18.7 (mean ± SD of 6 subjects) and 110.6 ± 27.8 (mean ± SD of 3 subjects) for 90 and 180 minutes of hypo-osmotic dialysis respec-

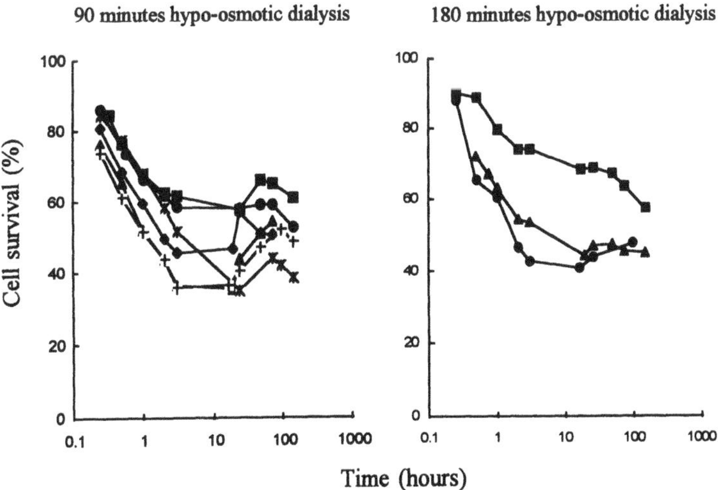

Figure 1. *In vivo* survival of unloaded carrier erythrocytes in 6 subjects injected with cells hypo-osmotically dialysed for 90 minutes and in 3 subjects injected with cells hypo-osmotically dialysed for 180 minutes. Results are expressed as a percentage of zero time values, calculated by extrapolation of the counts obtained for the first 3 hours after injection.

Table 1. Carrier erythrocyte *in vivo* survival results

Subject	Hypo-osmotic dialysis time (minutes)	Mean daily urinary exretion of label (%)	Cell survival (Days)	
			$t_{1/2}$	MCL
1	90	-	29	90.7
2		-	22	117.0
3		1.0	28	124.2
4		1.3	27	102.4
5		2.0	24	78.6
6		2.3	32	123.1
7	180	1.5	35	142.7
8		2.5	27	96.6
9		2.8	25	92.6

tively. The normal mean cell life is 110 days, ranging from 89 to 131 days. There were no differences in mean cell life using the two hypo-osmotic dialysis times ($p>0.5$).

3.2. Surface Counting

Surface counting demonstrated an initial loss of counts from the heart at both hypo-osmotic dialysis times. This coincided with an increase in splenic counts in three 90 minute hypo-osmotic dialysis cases and in one 180 minute hypo-osmotic dialysis case (Figure 2). These results show that the initial loss of labelled carrier erythrocytes from the circulation was due to sequestration by the spleen. There was no evidence of erythrocyte sequestration by the liver. The following increase in heart counts and decrease in splenic counts (in all cases) is consistent with a release of a proportion of the sequestered carrier erythrocytes back into the circulation, and accounts for the observed increase in circulating label (Figure 2).

3.3. Urinary Excretion

The mean daily urinary excretion of label was 1.7 ± 0.6% (mean ± SD of 4 subjects) and 2.3 ± 0.7% (mean ± SD of 3 subjects) for 90 minutes and 180 minutes of hypo-osmotic dialysis respectively (Table 1). There were no significant differences in excretion between the two hypo-osmotic dialysis times ($p>0.1$). These urinary excretions are well within the normal ^{51}Cr elution limits of 1.0 to 3.2% demonstrating that there was minimal intra vascular haemolysis of the labelled cells. This is supported by the fact that all label was cell-associated.

4. CONCLUSION

These *in vivo* survival results support the use of carrier erythrocytes as a sustained therapeutic drug and enzyme delivery and containment system. However, *in vivo* survival studies on therapeutic agent-loaded carrier erythrocytes are essential to ascertain that loading is not detrimental to carrier erythrocyte viability. The fact that the extended hypo-os-

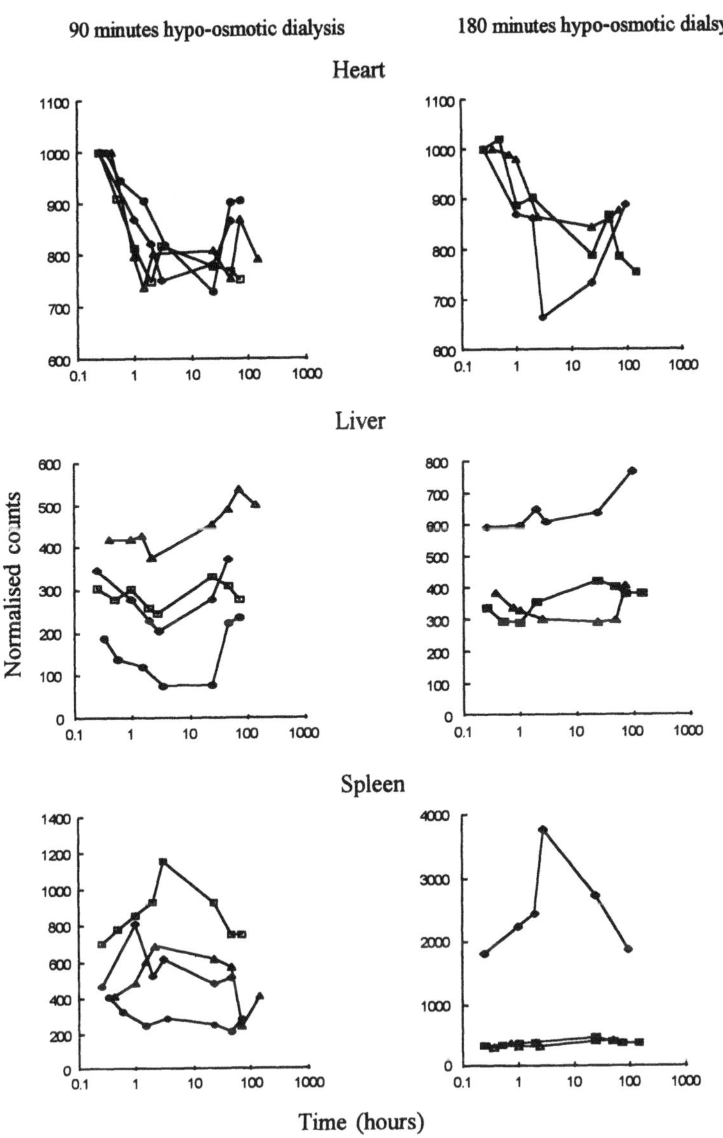

Figure 2. Normalised counts in heart, liver and spleen in 4 subjects injected with carrier erythrocytes hypo-osmotically dialysed for 90 minutes and in 3 subjects injected with carrier erythrocytes hypo-osmotically dialysed for 180 minutes.

motic dialysis period had no detrimental effect on cell survival is an important consideration where therapeutic agent entrapment is time dependent.

5. ACKNOWLEDGMENT

These studies were supported by the Wellcome Trust.

6. REFERENCES

Bax, B.E., Bain, M.D., Ward, C.P., Fensom, A.H. and Chalmers, R.A. The entrapment of mannose-terminated glucocerebrosidase (Alglucerase) in human carrier erythrocytes. Biochem. Soc. Trans. 24: 441S (1996a).

Bax, B.E., Fairbanks, D.L., Bain, M.D., Simmonds, H.A. and Chalmers, R.A. The entrapment of polyethylene glycol-bound adenosine deaminase (Pegademase) in human carrier erythrocytes. Biochem. Soc. Trans. 24: 442S (1996b).

Bax, B.E., Talbot, P.J., Bain, M.D., Parker-Williams, E.J. and Chalmers, R.A. *In vivo* survival of human carrier erythrocytes. Clin. Sci. 91:1P (1996c).

International Committee for Standardization in Haematology. Recommended methods for radioisotope red-cell survival studies. Br. J. Haematol. 45:659–666 (1980).

Sprandel, U., Hubbard, A.R. and Chalmers, R.A. Survival of 'carrier erythrocytes' in dogs. Clin. Sci. 59: 7P (1980).

Sprandel, U., Hubbard, A.R. and Chalmers, R.A. Towards enzyme therapy using carrier erythrocytes. J. Inher. Metab. Dis. 4:99–100 (1981).

THE ENTRAPMENT OF POLYETHYLENE GLYCOL-CONJUGATED ADENOSINE DEAMINASE (PEGADEMASE) AND NATIVE ADENOSINE DEAMINASE IN HUMAN CARRIER ERYTHROCYTES

Bridget E. Bax,[1] Lynette D. Fairbanks,[2] Murray D. Bain,[1]
H. Anne Simmonds,[2] and Ronald A. Chalmers[1]

[1]Paediatric Metabolism Unit
Department of Child Health
St George's Hospital Medical School
London, United Kingdom
[2]The Purine Research Laboratories
Guy's Hospital
London, United Kingdom

1. INTRODUCTION

Severe combined immunodeficiency (SCID) is a rare disorder with an incidence of 1:66 000. It is characterised by a defective humoral (hypogammaglobulinaemia) and cellular (lymphopenia) immunity and if untreated is severe and often lethal. Some 20% to 25% of SCID cases are due to a deficiency of adenosine deaminase (EC 3.5.4.4). Adenosine deaminase (ADA) is normally present in all mammalian cells and catalyses the deamination of adenosine and 2′-deoxyadenosine to inosine and 2′-deoxyinosine respectively for either salvage and re-utilisation or metabolism to uric acid and excretion. The major route of adenosine metabolism at physiological substrate levels is phosphorylation rather than deamination, this is because the K_m for adenosine kinase (EC 2.7.1.20) is lower than that of ADA. Adenosine in excess of physiological levels is degraded by ADA. The major source of 2′-deoxyadenosine is DNA turnover and the main route of its metabolism is deamination by ADA.

A deficiency in ADA results in a plasma accumulation of 2′-deoxyadenosine and a preferential phosphorylation of 2′-deoxyadenosine to deoxyadenosine triphosphate (dATP). dATP is unable to cross cell membranes and as a result, accumulates in high concentrations in rapidly dividing cells such as lymphocytes. The elevated cellular dATP concentrations are thought to impair lymphocyte differentiation and proliferation and thus

Erythrocytes as Drug Carriers in Medicine, edited by Sprandel and Way
Plenum Press, New York, 1997

prevent the effective functioning of the immune system. Lymphotoxicity has also been associated with the inhibition of the transmethylation enzyme, S-adenosylhomocysteine hydrolase by the accumulated 2′-deoxyadenosine (Simmonds, 1994; Herschfield and Mitchell, 1995).

The covalent attachment of polyethylene glycol to enzymes to enhance their circulation half-life and reduce immunogenicity has resulted in the production of the licensed pharmaceutical polyethylene glycol-conjugated adenosine deaminase (Pegademase). Pegademase provides an enzyme replacement therapy for ADA deficiency but is expensive due to high pharmaceutical production costs and rapid clearance from the vascular compartment (*in vivo* half-life of 3 to 6 days). Frequent infusions are required to maintain therapeutic plasma levels making treatment very invasive (Hershfield, 1993).

In this study we investigated the entrapment of Pegademase (molecular weight of 90 000 Daltons) in energy-replete carrier erythrocytes with the future aim of extending the *in vivo* enzyme half-life and maintaining therapeutic blood levels, thus reducing the frequency of therapeutic interventions and to substantially reduce the cost of enzyme therapy. The extent of Pegademase encapsulation using two different hypo-osmotic dialysis periods was determined. Carrier erythrocytes were also loaded with native ADA (molecular weight 33 500 Daltons) to investigate the effect of polyethylene glycol groups on the extent of enzyme entrapment.

2. METHODS

2.1. Preparation of Carrier Erythrocytes

Energy-replete carrier erythrocytes were prepared using a hypo-osmotic dialysis procedure (Sprandel, Hubbard and Chalmers, 1980; Sprandel, Hubbard and Chalmers; 1981). Seven volumes of washed and packed erythrocytes were mixed with 3 volumes of cold phosphate buffered saline (PBS) (136.89 mmol/l NaCl, 2.68 mmol/l KCl, 8.10 mmol/l Na_2HPO_4, 1.47 mmol/l KH_2PO_4, pH 7.4) containing varying concentrations of either Pegademase (Enzon, stock concentration 250 units/ml at 25°C) or native ADA from Calf intestinal mucosa (Sigma Chemical Co., stock concentration 1482 units/ml at 25°C). Five ml of this cell suspension were then placed into a 10 ml dialysis bag with a molecular weight cut-off of 12 000 Daltons. After sealing, the dialysis bag was placed into a container holding 150 ml hypo-osmotic buffer (5 mmol/l KH_2PO_4, 5 mmol/l K_2HPO_4, pH 7.4) and dialysed at 4°C with rotation at 6 rpm for 90 or 180 minutes with Pegademase or for 90 minutes with ADA. The lysed erythrocytes were resealed by transferring the dialysis bag to a container holding 150 ml PBS supplemented with 5 mmol/l adenosine, 5 mmol/l glucose and 5 mmol/l $MgCl_2$, pH 7.4 and continuing rotation at 6 rpm for 60 minutes at 37°C. Endogenous ADA activity was measured in controls prepared by lysing and re-sealing in the absence of Pegademase or ADA (unloaded carrier erythrocytes). The carrier erythrocytes were washed three times in 3 volumes iso-osmotic supplemented PBS with centrifugation at 100g for 15 minutes.

To control for binding of Pegademase and ADA to the outside of the erythrocyte membrane during enzyme-loaded carrier erythrocyte preparation, cells were dialysed with either Pegademase for 90 or 180 minutes, or ADA for 90 minutes at 4°C against iso-osmatic PBS(instead of hypo-osmotic buffer), followed by dialysis in supplemented PBS for 60 minutes at 37°C.

2.2. ADA and Pegademase Assay

Endogenous ADA activity and entrapped Pegademase and ADA activity were assayed by following the deamination of adenosine to inosine. Diluted and haemolysed carrier erythrocytes were incubated with 3.75 mmol/l adenosine in 100 mmol/l phosphate buffer for 1 hour. The reaction was stopped with 40% trichloroacetic acid, the excess of which was extracted from the supernatant with water-saturated diethyl ether. The reaction products were separated by HPLC using a Waters trimodular system with a Spherisorb ODS2 column and an isocratic tetrabutylammonium chloride and ammonium acetate buffer.

3. RESULTS

Figure 1 shows the entrapment of Pegademase and ADA as a function of enzyme units added to the dialysis bag. Logarithmic scales are used on both axes. In each case the amount of enzyme entrapped increased with added concentration. Doubling the hypo-osmotic time from 90 to 180 minutes resulted in a three-fold increase in Pegademase entrapment when less than 20 units of enzyme were added. This effect was abolished at enzyme concentrations greater than 20 units.

Entrapment of native ADA when a hypo-osmotic dialysis time of 90 minutes was used, was considerably higher than that of Pegademase at either 90 or 180 minutes (Bax et al.,1996). Using a total of 100 units per dialysis, ADA entrapment was 6-fold and 3.6-fold greater than that observed with Pegademase at 90 and 180 minutes respectively. These results suggest that the entrapment of Pegademase is limited by the polyethylene glycol groups.

Pegademase and ADA activities were not associated with cells that had been dialysed in iso-osmotic PBS, demonstrating that Pegademase and ADA do not bind to the outside of the erythrocyte membrane. The carrier erythrocyte-associated Pegademase and ADA thus represent entrapped enzyme.

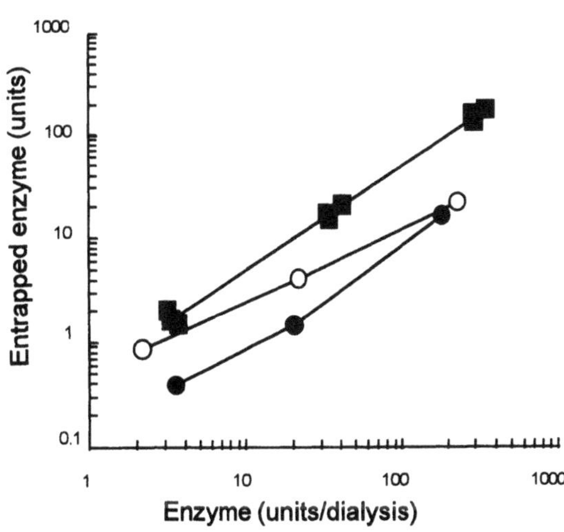

Figure 1. The entrapment of Pegademase and ADA by energy-replete carrier erythrocytes. Each point represents one dialysis experiment. ● Pegademase, 90 minutes of hypo-osmotic dialysis; ○ Pegademase, 180 minutes of hypo-osmotic dialysis; ■ ADA, 90 minutes of hypo-osmotic dialysis. One unit of activity is defined as the amount of enzyme required to convert 1 μmol of adenosine to inosine per minute at 37°C.

4. CONCLUSIONS

This study demonstrates a successful entrapment of a substantial proportion of free ADA and a smaller entrapment of Pegademase. The reasons for polyethylene glycol attachment are for prolonging circulation half-life, reducing immunogenity and prevention of ADA binding to ADA -complexing proteins. In the carrier erythrocyte model the attachment of polyethylene glycol becomes redundant, thus suggesting a potential therapeutic use of free ADA-loaded carrier erythrocytes in treating ADA deficiency.

5. ACKNOWLEDGMENT

These studies were supported by the Wellcome Trust.

6. REFERENCES

Bax, B.E., Fairbanks, D.L., Bain, M.D., Simmonds, H.A. and Chalmers, R.A. The entrapment of polyethylene glycol-bound adenosine deaminase (Pegademase) in human carrier erythrocytes. Biochem. Soc. Trans. 24: 442S (1996).

Herschfield, M.S. Enzyme replacement therapy of adenosine deaminase deficiency with polyethylene glycol-modified adenosine deaminase (PEG-ADA). Immunodefic. 4: 93–97 (1993).

Herschfield, M.S. and Mitchell, B.S. Immunodeficiency diseases caused by adenosine deaminase deficiency and purine nucleoside phosphorylase deficiency. In The Molecular and Metabolic Basis of Inherited Disease (ed. Scriver, C.R., Beaudet, A.L., Sly, W.S. and Valle, D.) Vol. II, pp1725–1768, McGraw-Hill, New York (1995).

Simmonds, H.A. Purine and pyrimidine disorders. In The Inherited Metabolic Diseases. (ed. Holton, J.B.) pp 297–349., Churchill Livingstone, Edinburgh (1994).

Sprandel, U., Hubbard, A.R. and Chalmers, R.A. Survival of 'carrier erythrocytes' in dogs. Clin. Sci. 59: 7P (1980).

Sprandel, U., Hubbard, A.R. and Chalmers, R.A. Towards enzyme therapy using carrier erythrocytes. J. Inher. Metab. Dis. 4:99–100 (1981).

5

USE OF ERYTHROCYTES AS A NEW ROUTE OF ADMINISTRATION OF FIBRINOLYTIC AGENTS

Preliminary Results

Benedicte Delahousse, Roger Kravtzoff, and Claude Ropars

Laboratoire de Biopharmacologie Transfusionnelle
INSERM U. 316 - C.R.T.S. - B.P. 2009
37020 Tours
France

1. INTRODUCTION

Red blood cells (RBCs) are easy to obtain, their cellular volume is large enough to load high quantities of active substances and their half-life is well defined. Due to their physiological role, they have access to most parts of the body. If transfusion rules are respected they are neither toxic nor immunogenic, and finally they are biodegradable. As largely demonstrated in the past, these properties allow them to be used as drug carriers in important pharmacological applications .

Many studies have been published concerning the use of erythrocytes as enzyme carriers. Several tentative experiments have been performed to load RBCs with therapeutic agents acting on coagulation mechanisms. This was the case for factors IX and X (Goldsmith et al. 1979), heparin (Eichleir et al. 1986), aspirin (Orekhova et al. 1990) and more recently brinase (Flynn et al. 1994). We evaluated the possibility to use human RBCs as fibrinolytic agent carriers with a new approach to long term venous thrombolytic therapy. Loaded erythrocytes could be administered by autotransfusion to prevent thrombosis in subjects with particular risk factors. Internalisation of fibrinolytic agents in red blood cells could be of value in terms of increased life span, protection against rapid inactivation by circulating antibodies, proteolytic degradation in the blood flow and use of lower dosages. Furthermore loaded erythrocytes could constitute a circulating reservoir of fibrinolytic agents acting only during a clotting process and being released *in situ* when the red blood cells spontaneously lysed within the clot fragment. Fibrinolytic agents could thus act during clot formation without the systemic activation of fibrinolysis, lowering the risk of haemorrhage.

Erythrocytes as Drug Carriers in Medicine, edited by Sprandel and Way
Plenum Press, New York, 1997

The aim of this study was to verify that, without important change in their physiologic and metabolic characteristics, red blood cells could internalise various fibrinolytic agents. Streptokinase (SK), urokinase (UK) or recombinant tissue plasminogen activator (t-PA) were internalised using a technique of hypotonic osmotic shock and their lytic effectiveness was evaluated. It was also necessary to ensure that there was no degradation of the fibrinolytic agents inside RBCs and that these loaded cells could act during clot formation without systemic fibrinolysis.

2. MATERIAL AND METHODS

2.1. Reagents and Controls

2.1.1 Fibrinolytics. - Streptokinase (Streptase®-Hoescht). 250,000 IU was purified from accompanying excipients using Sephadex G100 chromatography.

-Urokinase (Actosolve®-Hoescht). 600,000 IU.

-t-PA (Actilyse®-Boeringher Ingelheim). Freeze dried 20 mg

2.1.2 Internalisation Method. We used the small scale batch lysis-resealing internalisation method of DeLoach (1986), for human and mouse RBCs.

2.1.3. Fibrinolytic Enzymatic Activity. - We used the chromogenic method derived of Friberger and Knös (1980), using purified plasminogen and chromogen S2251.

-For comparison, the various fibrinolytic concentrations were standardised using a common activity arbitrary unit: 1 AU = variation of 1 unit optical density/mn.

*Urokinase: 1 AU= 690 IU or 0.384 mg of lyophilised UK.

*Streptokinase: 1 AU= 0.054 mg of lyophilised SK

*t-PA: 1 AU= 0.10 mg lyophilised t-PA

2.1.4. Fibrinolytic Molecule Radiolabeling. UK and t-PA were labeled with ^{125} Iodide using chloramin T.

2.1.5. Fibrinolytic Activity on Standardised Clots. Human RBCs were collected using citrate 45 mmol. l^{-1}, Na_2HPO_4 15 mmol l^{-1}, glucose 130 mmol l^{-1} , pH 7.4 (CPD, Bruneau France) as anticoagulant. RBCs were suspended at 50% haematocrit in compatible plasma. Clot formation was induced by introducing calcium chloride 0.117 mol l^{-1} in RBCs suspension. Clots were formed using normal control or treated RBCs.

Clot formation parameters or total lysis time in the presence of fibrinolytics were evaluated using thromboelastogram measurements (TEG).

2.2. Evaluation of Plasmatic Parameters of Fibrinolysis

In the various samples, the following measurement methods were used:

-Fibrinogen: automated Von Claus method.

-Plasminogen: automated chromogenic method using H-D-Nva-CHA-lys-pNA (paranitro aniline reagent - Chromotimer® Behring).

-Alpha 2 antiplasmin: similar automated chromogenic method using standardised plasmin reagent.

-D-dimers: dosage of specific fibrin degradation products using the immunoenzymatic kit (Stago) with a specific monoclonal antibody anti-D-dimers.

2.3 Internalisation Process in Human RBCs

The protocol of DeLoach (1986) was used with the following parameters:

-Urokinase: UK concentration at 5, 2.5, 1.25 and 0.25 mg/ml corresponding to respectively 13.5, 6.75, 3.375 and 0.675 AU/ml were used for internalisation. The dialysis time was 45 mn or 60 mn.

-Streptokinase: SK 7.25, 21.75 and 50.75 AU/ml during a dialysis time of 45 mn.

-t-PA: 0.25 AU/ml was dialysed during 45 mn

3. RESULTS

3.1. Internalisation Parameters

The various internalisation yields obtained for a dialysis time of 45 mn are presented in the Table 1.

In the Table 2 are presented the haematological parameters of fibrinolytics-loaded and control RBCs

3.2. Total Lysis Time for UK and SK Free and Internalised in Human RBCs

The fibrinolytics-loaded RBCs were washed and suspended in a compatible plasma at 50% haematocrit. Controls RBCs were treated in the same way. After introduction of calcium chloride in the suspension, the total lysis time for clotted RBCs suspensions containing various doses of free or internalised fibrinolytics was measured using TEG. The results are presented on Fig. 1 and 2, respectively for UK and SK.

3.3. Evolution of Plasmatic Parameters of Fibrinolysis

Fibrinolytics circulating or introduced in a blood sample, in the absence of any clot formation, activate plasminogen to plasmin. Consequently, the concentration of plasminogen decreases, alpha 2 antiplasmin and fibrinogen are consumed and fibrin degradation products (D-dimers) are formed. These "adverse effects" are responsible of the haemorrhage risk of the classical treatments by fibrinolytics. On the contrary, after clotting, the decrease of plasminogen, of alpha 2 antiplasmin and the production of D-dimers are the signs of an efficient fibrinolysis.

Table 1. Internalisation yield of fibrinolytics in RBCs (dialysis time 45 mn;)

	UK	SK	t-PA
Dose used	2.5 mg/ml -6.75 AU/ml	7.25 AU/ml	0.25 AU/ml -2.5 mg/ml
Internalisation yield	41 ± 8%	31± 8%	30± 6%

Table 2. Haematological parameters of fibrinolytics-loaded and controls RBCs (dialysis time 45 mn)

	MCV	MCHC	MCHC
Controls n=15	90.4±1.3	31.9±1.1	29.6±0.6
UK (6.75 AU/ml) n=2	78.6±1.9	29.6±0.3	23.3±0.8
SK (7.25 AU/ml) n=9	72±2.9	33.3±1.6	23.9±1.1
t-PA (0.25 AU/ml) n=3	80.6±5.1	31.4±0.3	24.6±0.6

We have controlled that UK internalised in RBCs did not produce the adverse effects observed with free UK in non clotted samples at 37°C. The dose used was 0.45 AU/ml at 100% haematocrit corresponding to 0.225 AU/ml in a 50% plasma sample.

The results are presented on Fig. 3. They are expressed as the ratio versus the values obtained for a control sample which did not contained UK and submitted to the same protocol (incubation at 37°C, clotted or non clotted).

3.4. *In Vitro* Stability of Fibrinolytics Internalised in RBCs

After internalisation treatment, human RBCs were washed, suspended in compatible plasma at 40% haematocrit and incubated at 37°C during 48 h. The percentages of fibrinolytic activity were expressed versus the initial values. For comparison, the variation of haemoglobin percentage after RBCs washing was also evaluated to detect a possible haemolysis of the RBCs containing the fibrinolytics. The results for a period of 24 h are expressed on the Fig. 4.

3.5. *In Vivo* Stability in Mouse RBCs

To evaluate the *in vivo* stability of fibrinolytics loaded in RBCs, 6.75 AU/ml of UK and 15 AU/ml of SK have been internalised in mouse erythrocytes using the same proto-

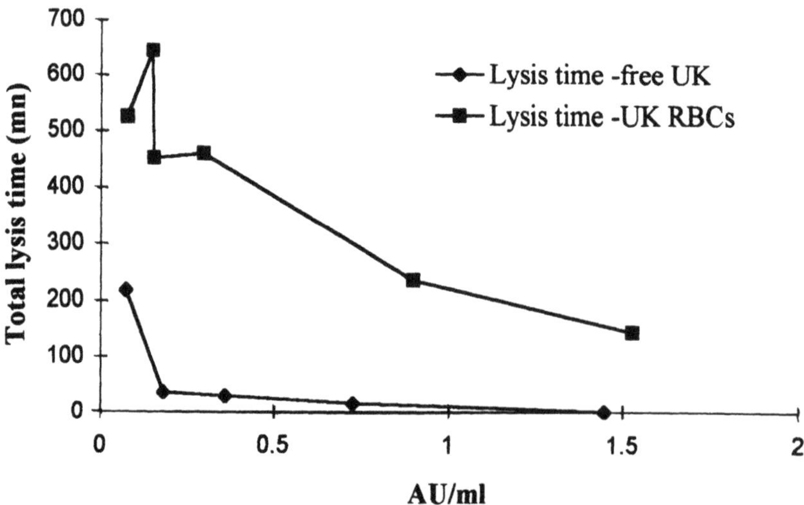

Figure 1. Evaluation of the total lysis time obtained for free and internalised Urokinase at various doses.

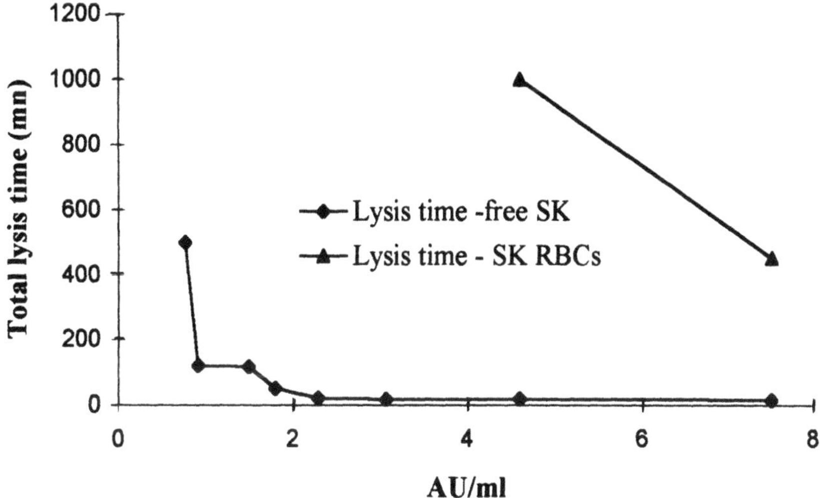

Figure 2. Evaluation of the total lysis time obtained for free and internalised Streptokinase at various doses.

col as for human RBCs. The internalisation yields were lower than for human RBCs, respectively 18.7 % for UK and 10.7% for SK. The final concentration in packed RBCs, calculated for a 100% haematocrit, were 2.04 AU/ml for UK and 3.5 AU/ml for SK. After ^{51}Cr labeling, the RBCs were injected at the tail of mice (200µl at 40% Ht). The radioactivity and fibrinolytic activities were measured at 10 mn, 1, 3, 6, 18, 24 and 48h. Each measurement was performed in triplicate.

For UK, no activity was detected after 10 mn, showing a very rapid degradation. For SK, 40% activity was recovered after 1h and the lytic activity disappeared at 18h. Such decrease in the circulating activity was not related to the disappearance of transformed mouse RBCs as the half life determined using ^{51}Cr radioactivity were respectively 13.5 and 13.3 days for UK and SK.

The comparison of the stability of SK *in vitro* (human) and *in vivo* (mouse) is presented on Fig. 5.

4. DISCUSSION

These results show that the three fibrinolytic molecules we have studied may be introduced in human RBCs with yields similar to that previously observed for molecules having a similar molecular weight. The cellular characteristics were also identical to that previously published for other molecules.

The lytic properties of the fibrinolytics after internalisation in human RBCs, as studied using tromboelastogram recording, are maintained *in vitro* for several hours. When internalised, the fibrinolytics did not eliminate the first period of clot formation. The comparison of the total lysis time for free or internalised fibrinolytics shows that at equivalent concentration the internalisation process increases the period of clot lysis. This may be explained by a partial lysis of the cells containing the enzyme or to a partial retention of the drug inside the membranous ghost. In the case of intracellular fibrinolytics, the increased total lysis time could be due to the fact that the molecules are only progressively

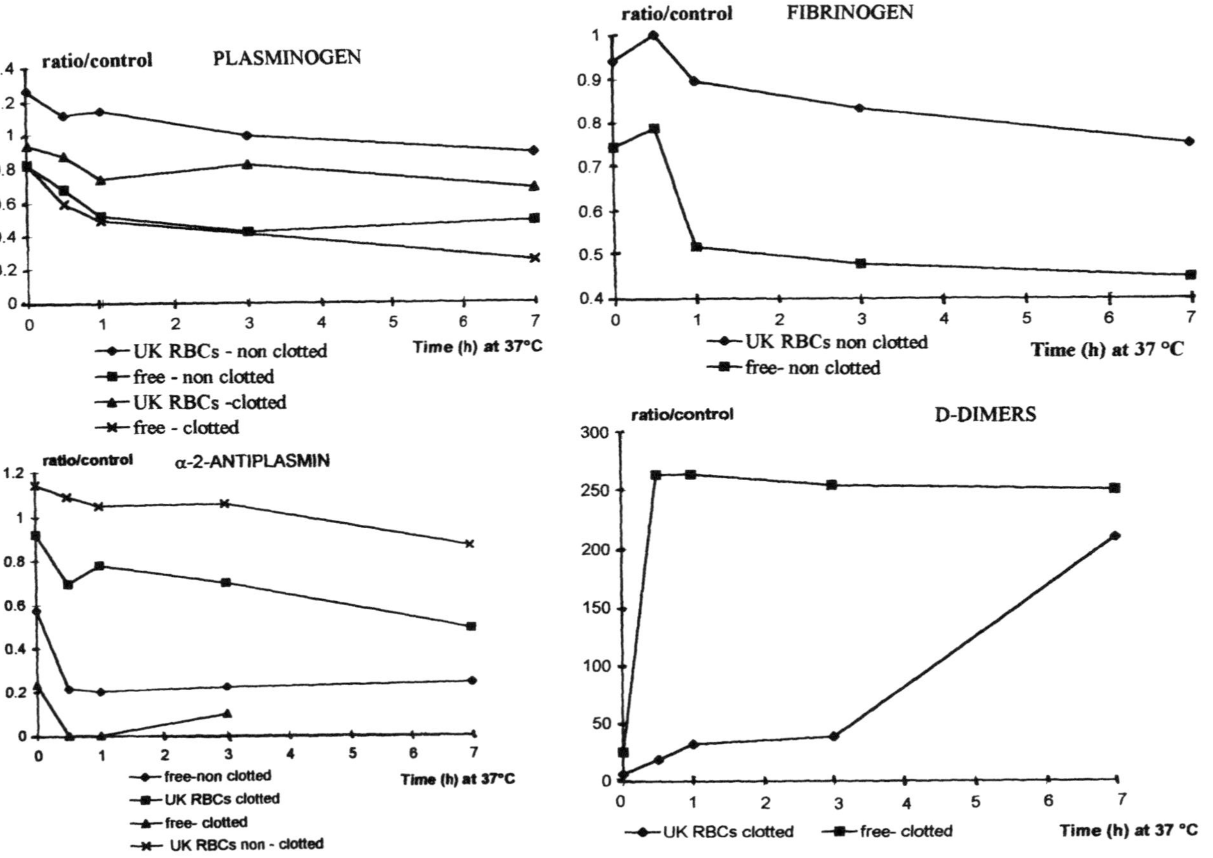

Figure 3. Evolution of plasmatic fibrinolysis parameters before and after clotting for blood suspensions containing Urokinase 0.45 AU/ml. Results are expressed as a ratio versus the value obtained for a control, without UK, submitted to the same treatment (37°C, clotted or non clotted)

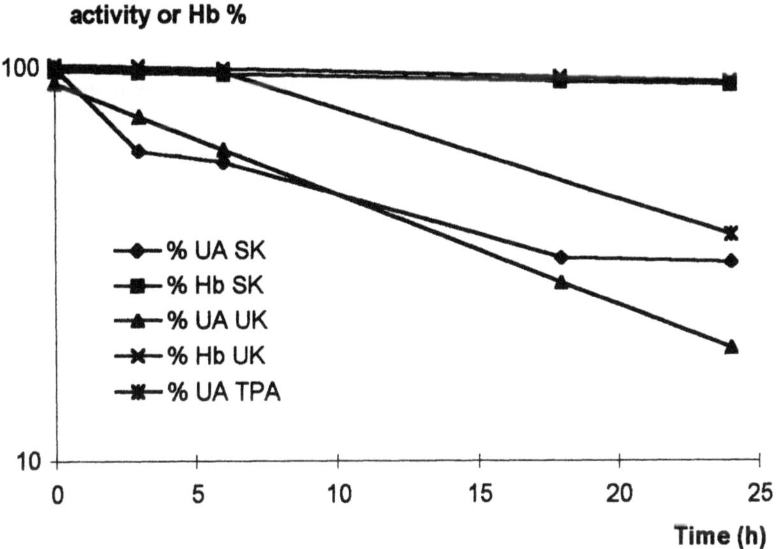

Figure 4. In vitro stability of three fibrinolytics internalized in RBC's (human). Variations % of enzymatic activities or of haemoglobin in washed RBC's.

liberated in the clot after the destruction of the cellular carrier . The activation of plasminogen is thus progressive but sufficient to obtain the lysis of the clot. This could explain that, contrary to external fibrinolytics, the drugs internalised in RBCs did not inhibit the clot formation.

The comparison of Fig. 1 and 2 show that the lytic activity of UK is more important than that of SK at equivalent concentrations expressed in arbitrary activity units (AU/ml). For extracellular fibrinolytics, a lysis time of 60 mn was observed for 0.25 AU/ml of UK and 1.25 AU/ml of SK. A total inhibition of coagulation was observed for 1.25 AU/ml of

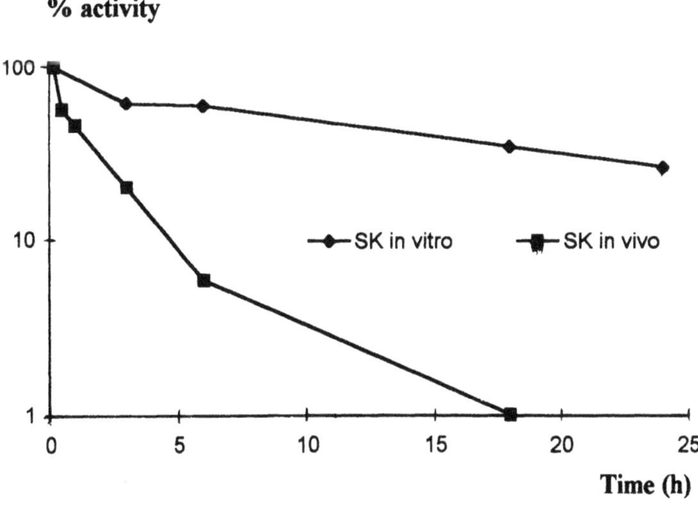

Figure 5. Comparison of the stabilty in vitro (human) and in vivo (mouse) of Streptokinase internalised in RBC's.

UK and 6.5 AU/ml of SK. These results may be explained by the differences in the mechanism of action of these two molecules. UK acts directly on plasminogen. SK needs a first step of complex formation with plasminogen. This complex will then activate another molecule of plasminogen. When the fibrinolytics were internalised, the phenomenon seams to be increased. For a concentration of UK (1.5 AU/ml) inducing the lysis of the clot in 150 mn, no activity was observed for SK. The highest dose of SK (10.5 AU/ml) induces the clot lysis in 500 mn; this time was obtained for UK with a 40 times lower dose (0.25 AU/ml).

At the doses used, the internalised fibrinolytics did not produce the systemic fibrinolysis observed with free drugs. As shown on the Fig. 3, the non clotted samples of UK remain similar to the control (ratio = 1) for 7 h. The enzyme was not liberated from the RBCs without clotting. Inversely, the free enzyme activates immediately the plasminogen, decreases the alpha 2 antiplasmin factor concentration and liberates fibrin degradation products (D-dimers). After clotting, intracellular UK was liberated and a progressive fibrinolysis was evidenced, notably with the decrease in alpha 2 antiplasmin and D-dimers production. This last parameter was similar to that obtained with free drug after 7h.

The stability measurements *in vitro* and *in vivo* have shown a rapid destruction of the enzymes internalised in RBCs. This was evidenced from the enzymatic activity degradation which was much more rapid than the *in vitro* RBCs haemolysis or the *in vivo* life span of the carrier. This may be explained by an intracellular oxidation or proteolytic degradation. UK and t-PA are particularly labile. SK is the most resistant molecule. Unfortunately, these results are not in favour of our preliminary objective that was to obtain a sustained transport of fibrinolytics in RBCs carriers, with the molecules we have studied. However, such result may be expected using modified and stabilised molecules, for example using PEG coating, to improve the proteolytic stability. Other molecules are also presently existing with fibrinolytic activity, which could be more stable when internalised in RBCs.

5. REFERENCES

DeLoach J.R. Carrier Erythrocytes. Medicinal. Res. Rev. (1986) ***6***: 487–504.

Eichler H.G., Schneider W., Raberger G., Bacher S. and Pabinger I. Erythrocytes as carriers of heparin. Res. Exp. Med. (1986) ***186***: 407–412.

Flynn G., Hackett T.J., McHale L. and McHale A.P. Encapsulation of the thrombolytic enzyme, brinase, in photosensitized erythrocytes: a novel thrombolytic system based on photodynamc activation. J. Photochem. and Photobiol.(1994) ***26***: 193–196.

Friberger P. and Knös M. Functional assays of the components of the fibrinolytic system using a plasmin sensitive substrate. A review. In Linjnen H.R., Collen D. and Verstraete M. Ed; Synthetic substrates in coagulation blood assays. (1980) 73–91. Nijhof M. Pub. The Hague, Boston, London.

Goldsmith J.C., Roer M. E.S. and Orringer E.P. A new treatment strategy for hemophilia: Incorporation of factor IX into red cell ghosts. Amer. J. Hematol. (1979) ***7***: 119–125.

Orekhova N.M., Akchurin R.S., Belayev A.A., Smirnov M.D., Ragimov S.E. and Orekhov A.N. Local prevention of thrombosis in animal arteries by means of magnetic targeting of aspirin-loaded red cells. Thrombosis Res. (1990) ***57***: 611–616.

6

SYNTHESIS, CHARACTERIZATION, AND ERYTHROCYTE ENCAPSULATION OF AN AZIDOTHYMIDINE HOMODINUCLEOTIDE

Marco Giovine,[1] Sonia Scarfi,[1] Anna Gasparini,[1] Enrico Millo,[1] Gianluca Damonte,[1] Antonio De Flora,[1] Mauro Magnani,[2] Alessandra Fraternale,[2] Luigia Rossi,[2] Rosamund Williams,[3] and Umberto Benatti[1]

[1]Institute of Biochemistry
University of Genoa
Viale Benedetto XV/1
16132 Genoa, Italy
[2]Institute of Biochemistry "Giogio Fornaini"
University of Urbino
Via Saffi 2
61029 Urbino, Italy
[3]Lepetit Research Center
Gerenzano
21040 Varese
Italy

1. SUMMARY

A new nucleoside analogue, di(thymidine-3′-azido-2′,3′-dideoxy-D-riboside)-5′-5′-p^1-p^2-pyrophosphate ($AZTp_2AZT$), was designed and synthesized to overcome some limitations of conventional antiretroviral chemotherapy based upon nucleoside analogues (AZT, ddC, ddI). Indeed, the triphosphorylated form of these nucleoside analogues is able to inhibit the infectivity and replication of Human Immunodeficiency Virus (HIV-1), but the main problems in the use of these drugs concern their limited phosphorylation in some cells (e.g., macrophages) and their cytotoxic side effects. $AZTp_2AZT$ was encapsulated in human erythrocytes according to a conservative procedure of hypotonic shock-isotonic resealing and reannealing and showed a remarkable stability and a slow conversion to 5′-monophosphate (AZT-MP) and to AZT. This azidothymidine homodinucleotide seems to have chemical and biochemical properties enabling its profitable utilization in the erythrocyte-encapsulated form.

Erythrocytes as Drug Carriers in Medicine, edited by Sprandel and Way
Plenum Press, New York, 1997

2. INTRODUCTION

Nucleoside analogues, such as Azidothymidine (AZT), dideoxycytidine (ddC) and dideoxyinosine (ddI), are the most common drugs for the treatment of HIV-1 infection. To be pharmacologically active, the antiviral nucleoside analogues must first be phosphorylated by cellular kinases[3,8], but these enzymes usually have low levels in quiescent cells[6,7]. Moreover, AZT, ddC and ddI have a low permeability through cerebrospinal fluid and a low half-life in plasma[14]. Accordingly, high dosages and frequent administrations are necessary to obtain therapeutic efficacy, with consequent enhancement of toxicity for the organism.

$AZTp_2AZT$ (Fig. 1) was proposed to overcome these side effects and eventually to improve the therapeutic use of AZT by means of engineered erythrocytes[1,11]. This proposal stemmed, among other considerations, by the fact that properly engineered erythrocytes can improve the therapeutic activity of cytotoxic drugs, as already demonstrated with antitumor molecules such as Doxorubicin[15] and 5-Fluoro-2′-deoxyuridine[4]. In principle, there are two ways of employing erythrocytes as carriers of $AZTp_2AZT$. One is the use of autologous erythrocytes for direct targeting of the homodinucleotide to macrophages[11], thereby allowing a phosphorylated derivative of AZT, as a relevant pharmacologically active species of azidothymidine, to reach a selected site of HIV infection. The second one is the internalization in circulating, i.e. non-targeted red cells of $AZTp_2AZT$ as a prodrug, susceptible to be metabolically converted by endogenous erythrocyte enzymes to membrane-releasable active AZT[1].

3. MATERIALS AND METHODS

3.1. Synthesis and Characterization of $AZTp_2AZT$ (Fig. 1)

AZT-MP was synthesized and characterized as previously described.[10] AZT-MP tri-*n*-octilammonium salt was prepared by dissolving 0.25 mmol of AZT-MP-Na salt in 50% aqueous methanol and the solution was eluted through 1 g of Dowex 50W-X8 (pyridinium form). The eluate was dried under reduced pressure and the residue was resuspended in 3 ml of methanol and 0.45 ml of tri-*n*-octylammine. The mixture was stirred for 30 min at 25°C and vacuum dried. The residue was suspended in 2 ml of N,N-dimethylformamide and dried under reduced pressure. The latter procedure was repeated three times.

The residue was suspended in 4.5 ml of dioxane, 0.2 ml of diphenylchlorophosphate and 0.3 ml of tri-*n*-butylamine and the solution was stirred for 3h at room temperature and dried.

n-hexane (16 ml) was added, with vigorous shaking and the mixture left for 30 min in ice. Then it was centrifuged at 1,000 rpm for 5 min, the *n*-hexane was removed, the residue was dissolved in 2 ml of dioxane and vacuum dried and P^1-AZT-5′-P^2-diphenyl pyrophosphate was obtained.

P^1-AZT-5′-P^2-diphenyl pyrophosphate (0.25 mmol) was then dissolved in 1.8 ml of anhydrous pyridine and added to 0.25 mmol of the AZT-MP tri-*n*-octylammonium salt, prepared as above, together with 0.32 ml of hexamethylphosphotriamide. The mixture was dried under reduced pressure; afterwards, 0.4 ml of anhydrous pyridine was added to the residue and the resulting solution was stirred for 24 h at 25°C and then vacuum dried. The residue was suspended in 6 ml of H_2O, the pH was adjusted to 8.0 with 1 M NaOH, and the mixture was extracted three times with 6 ml of diethyl ether. The lower aqueous layer,

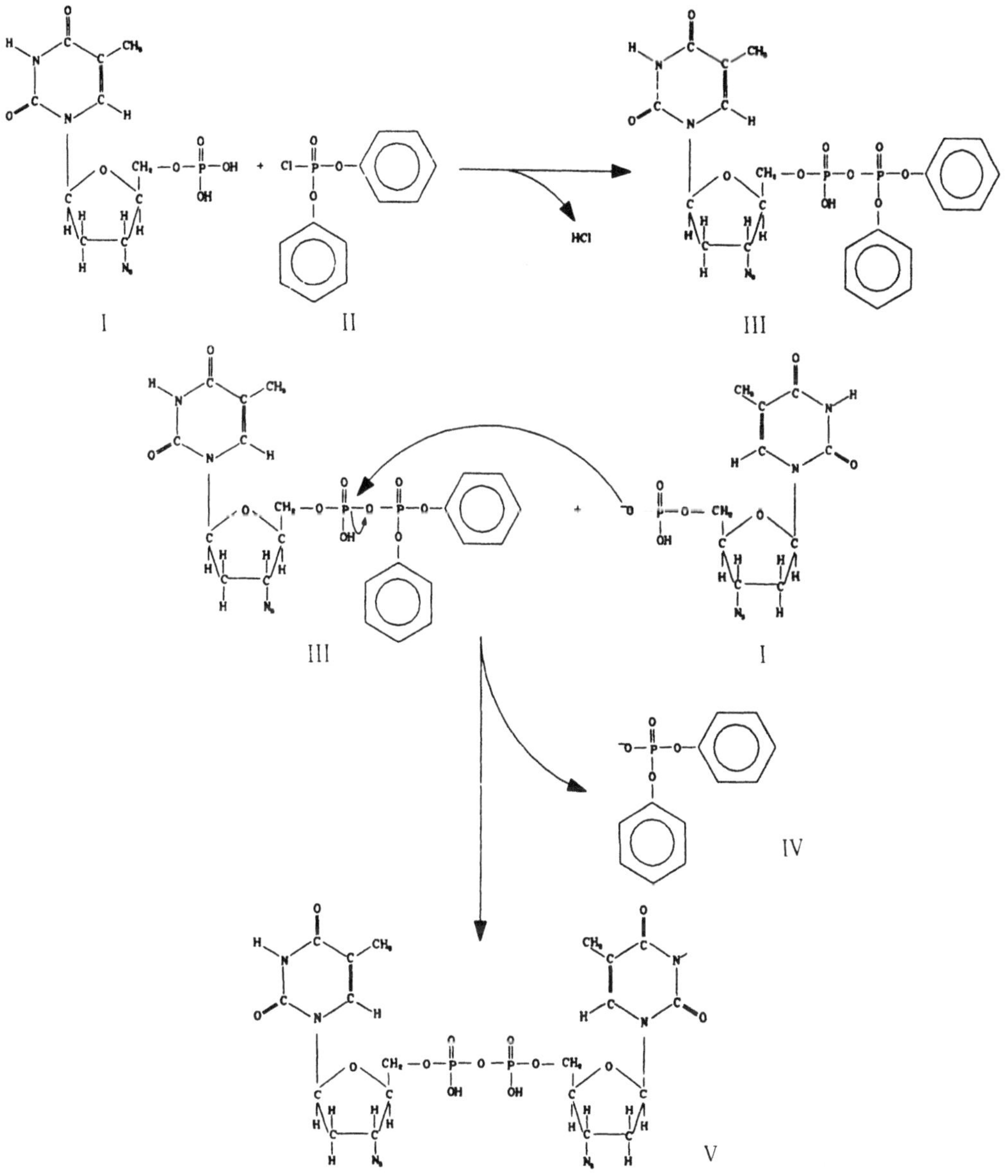

I II III

III I

IV

V

Figure 1. Flow sheet of synthesis of azidothymidine homodinucleotide. I. AZT-MP; II. diphenylchlorophosphate; III. P[1]-AZT-5′-P[2]-diphenyl pyrophosphate; IV. diphenylphosphate; V. $AZTp_2AZT$.

recovered by centrifugation, was then submitted to HPLC fractionation in 1-ml aliquots. A Bio-Sil C_{18} HL 90–10 reverse phase column (Bio-Rad; 210x10 mm, 10 μm particle size) was used. Elution was carried out stepwise with aqueous ethanol at increasing concentrations as follows: 3% (vol/vol) for 7 min, 5% for 10 min, 15% for 15 min, 100% for 16 min and the column was re-equilibrated again at 3% for 25 min at a constant flow of 6 ml/min. The eluted compounds were detected by a Shimadzu SPD-M6A photodiode array detector set at 260 nm. The nucleotide eluted at 11 min was lyophilized and submitted to chemical analyses.

Mass spectra were acquired in negative ion mode using a single quadrupole Hewlett-Packard Engine 5989A equipped with an electrospray ion source (ESPI-MS). Scan acquisition ranged in an interval including the expected molecular masses.

The ^1H NMR spectrum was recorded at 200 MHz in the temperature range from 20°C to 30°C on a Varian Gemini spectrometer in ^2H_2O.

3.2. $AZTp_2AZT$ stability in intact erythrocytes

Human erythrocytes were loaded with $AZTp_2AZT$ using the procedure of hypotonic hemolysis-isotonic resealing and reannealing[5,15] with some modifications. Briefly, washed and packed erythrocytes (83% Hematocrit) were dialyzed against 70 vol. of hemolysing buffer (5 mM Na_2HPO_4 supplemented with 4 mM $MgCl_2$, pH 7.2, 26 mOsm) for 30 min at 4° C under gentle rotation. Successively, 12 mM $AZTp_2AZT$ was added inside the dialysis bag and the dialysis was protracted for 15 additional min under the same conditions. Resealing was carried out by dialysing erythrocytes for 40 min at 4° C against phosphate-saline buffer pH 7.4, supplemented with 10 mM glucose and adenosine, 310 mOsm. Drug-loaded erythrocytes were extracted with perchloric acid as reported[2]. $AZTp_2AZT$ determination in neutralized extract was carried out using a 5 µm, 100 x 4,6 mm ODS-Hypersil C_{18} reverse-phase column (Hewlett-Packard). Solvent A was 0.1 M KH_2PO_4 containing 5 mM tetra-*n*-butylammonium (pH 4.9); solvent B was solvent A containing 40% (vol/vol) methanol. The solvent program was a linear gradient (at a flow rate of 0.4 ml/min) starting at 100% solvent A and increasing to 100% solvent B in 30 min. The various compounds were detected by a Hewlett-Packard 1040A diode array spectrophotometric detector set at 260 nm. The elution time of $AZTp_2AZT$ was 31 min.

4. RESULTS

4.1. Chemical Synthesis and Characterization of $AZTp_2AZT$

$AZTp_2AZT$ was synthesized as described above; the purification resulted in the salt-free compound with a 99.1% purity (HPLC) and the final yield of the process was 60%

Characterization of intermediates and of final compound was performed by ESPI-MS on a quadrupole instrument. Electrospray analysis allows to obtain spectra in a non-destructive mode, producing essentially molecular ions. When phosphate groups are present in a molecule, also sodium or potassium adducts can be detected.

The mass spectrum of the purified product of synthesis showed a molecular ion at m/z 675.9, consistent with the $[M-H]^-$ ion of the expected $AZTp_2AZT$ molecule (Fig. 2). The minor peak at m/z 697.7 corresponds to the $[M-2H+Na]^-$ ion of the same molecule. The NMR spectrum (Fig. 3) showed the most significant chemical shifts at 1.639 δppm ($-CH_3$), 2,225 δppm (-O-CH2), 3,943 δppm (broad 1′-CH and 2′-CH2), 4,275 δppm (3′-CH), 5,955 δppm (4′-CH) and 7.439 δppm (aromatic proton 6-CH). Taken together, these properties are consistent with the structure expected from the above described procedure of synthesis.

4.2. Stability of $AZTp_2AZT$ into Erythrocytes

Encapsulation of $AZTp_2AZT$ under the specific conditions described in the "Materials and Methods" section, yielded a final intraerythrocytic concentration of 4mM (Ta-

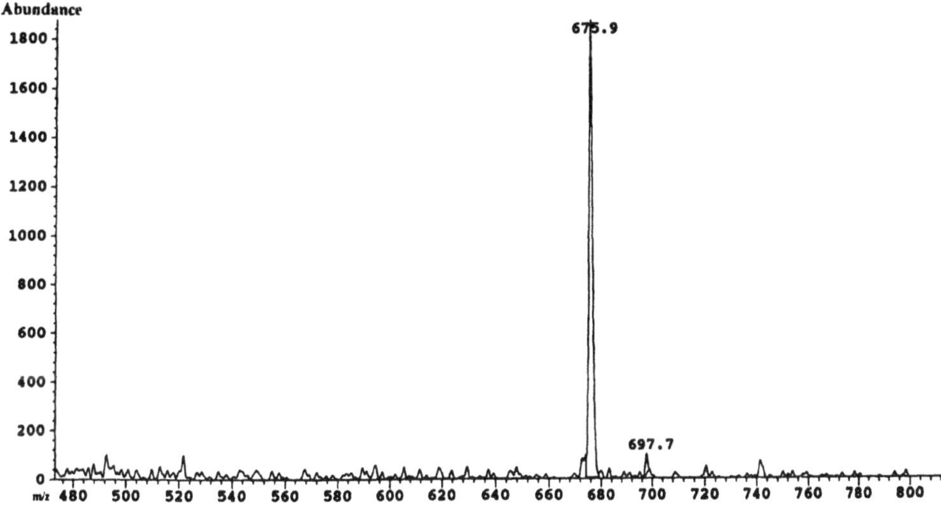

Figure 2. Mass spectrum of the synthesized molecule (from Magnani et al., 1996, modified)

ble 1), without any appreciable alteration of erythrocyte morphology and metabolic properties (not shown).

This concentration, resulting from adequate upgrading of the usual entrapment procedure, was deliberately selected to test the efficiency of the loaded erythrocytes as bioreactors competent to the release of azidothymidine[1]. To this purpose, engineered red blood cells were incubated in sterile conditions at a 10% hematocrit in autologous plasma .

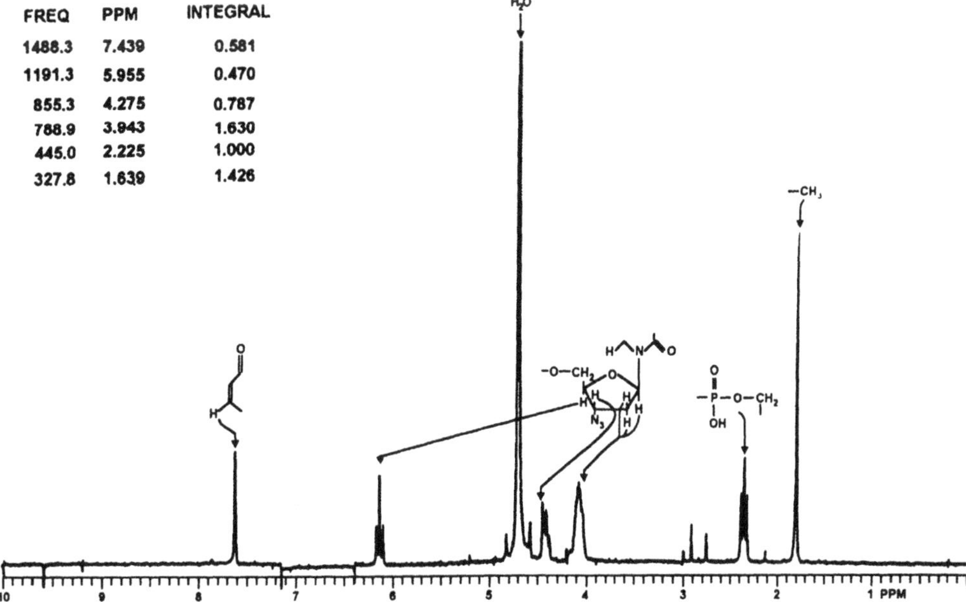

FREQ	PPM	INTEGRAL
1488.3	7.439	0.581
1191.3	5.955	0.470
855.3	4.275	0.787
788.9	3.943	1.630
445.0	2.225	1.000
327.8	1.639	1.426

Figure 3. NMR spectrum of the synthesized molecule.

Table 1. Concentration of $AZTp_2AZT$ and its metabolites into human red blood cells (expressed in nmoles/ml packed cells)

Time (hrs)	$AZTp_2AZT$	AZTMP	AZT
0	4,100	40	-
2	3,900	90	-
6	2,900	650	600
24	1,800	930	100

Table 1 shows the good stability of the compound (40% was still present into erythrocytes after 24 hours). It was evident that $AZTp_2AZT$ metabolism consisted in the production of AZTMP and AZT and that the latter metabolite was released in plasma as shown in Table 2.

The presence of small amounts of $AZTp_2AZT$ and AZT-MP in plasma was partially due to a low extent of hemolysis and to a direct release of AZT-MP across the erythrocyte membrane[10].

5. DISCUSSION

The design and build-up of a pharmacologically active new molecule require a careful and multi-faceted study on the specific cell targets and on the enzymatic pathways involved in drug metabolism. This project started from the need to synthesize a prodrug of azidothymidine suitable to protect different cell types like lymphocytes and macrophages from retroviral infection. We reasoned that, due to versatility of prodrug-loaded erythrocytes in behaving either as macrophage-targeted carriers[9] or as circulating bioreactors, encapsulation of such prodrug in red cells could provide in principle the advantages of a combination chemotherapy.

Central to the design of the novel azidothymidine homodinucleotide ($AZTp_2AZT$) reported earlier[11] and in this paper, is its susceptibility to dinucleotide pyrophosphatase activity. This enzyme, already identified and partially characterized in red cells[16], could catalyze the intraerythrocytic formation of AZT-MP, which has been previously reported to be a good precursor of azidothymidine[10]. Accordingly, the sequential operation of dinucleotide pyrophosphatase and of 5′-nucleotidase should ensure a sustained output of azidothymidine from $AZTp_2AZT$-loaded red cells.

Table 2. Concentration of $AZTp_2AZT$ and its metabolites in human plasma (expressed in nmoles/ml) (from Benatti et al., modified)

Time (hrs)	$AZTp_2AZT$	AZTMP	AZT
0	4.49	21.94	4.6
2	3.75	28.21	14.42
6	5.27	24.68	62.43
24	5.34	67.11	355.78

On the other hand, dinucleotide pyrophosphatase might play an essential role also in the macrophage compartment by converting $AZTp_2AZT$ to two molecules of AZT-MP, thereby overcoming the poor activity of macrophages to phosphorylate nucleoside analogues like azidothymidine[12,13]. In this case, an obvious requirement is that the encapsulated $AZTp_2AZT$ escapes complete intraerythrocytic degradation in order to reach the target macrophages in adequate amounts to be activated therein by conversion to the retroviral reverse transcriptase inhibitors, mostly to AZT 5′-triphosphate (AZT-TP).

Therefore, the interplay between erythrocyte and macrophage dinucleotide pyrophosphatases seems to be essential in the choice of the $AZTp_2AZT$-loaded red cells as macrophage-targeted systems or as circulating azidothymidine-releasing devices. The data reported in Table 1 and 2 indicate that the metabolic machinery of human erythrocytes (i.e., pyrophosphatase and 5′-nucleotidase) is competent to sustained production and output of azidothymidine. It should be noticed that these results were obtained following erythrocyte over-loading of $AZTp_2AZT$, as compared with earlier findings[1]. This performance of $AZTp_2AZT$-loaded erythrocytes is reminiscent of a previously reported intraerythrocytic two-step pathway resulting in the release of 5-fluoro-2′-deoxyuridine from human red cells loaded with a novel dimeric fluoropyrimidine molecule[5].

However, since the time required to induce phagocytosis of $AZTp_2AZT$-loaded and opsonized erythrocytes is shorter than that resulting in substantial $AZTp_2AZT$ consumption, the targeting to macrophages too is certainly possible, as previously demonstrated[11]. Accordingly, withdrawal of autologous erythrocytes followed by $AZTp_2AZT$ encapsulation might allow both lymphocytes and macrophages to be protected from HIV infection, by using both an unperturbed and an opsonized sample of the $AZTp_2AZT$-loaded erythrocytes, respectively.

Although the reported procedure of synthesis of $AZTp_2AZT$ was developed to build-up the homodinucleotide of azidothymidine, it can be properly modified in order to obtain other homodinucleotides representing different combinations of nucleoside analogues (e.g., ddC, ddA and ddI). In addition, such procedure seems to be suitable to obtain atypical heterodinucleotide structures based on 5′,5′-pyrophosphates of different chemotherapeutic agents, e.g. azidothymidine and acyclovir. Also in these cases, susceptibility of the new potential prodrug molecules to dinucleotide pyrophosphatase is the key requirement to trigger cell-specific bioactivation.

6. ACKNOWLEDGMENTS

This study was supported by the Italian Ministry of Health, Istituto Superiore di Sanità, Progetto AIDS, and by Gruppo Lepetit S.p.A., Lainate (Milan), Italy.

7. REFERENCES

1. Benatti, U., Giovine, M., Damonte, G., Gasparini, A., Scarfi, S., De Flora, A., Fraternale, A., Rossi, L. and Magnani, M. Azidothymidine homodinucleotide-loaded erythrocytes as bioreactors for slow delivery of the antiretroviral drug azidothymidine. Biochem. Biophys. Res. Commun. 220, 20–25, 1996.
2. Beutler E; Red Cells Metabolism. A manual of Biochemical methods. Grune&Stratton, Orlando, 1984.
3. De Clercq, E. Basic approaches to anti-retroviral treatment. J. AIDS 4, 207–218, 1991.
4. De Flora, A., Zocchi, E., Polvani, C. and Benatti, U. Conversion of encapsulated 5-fluoro-2′-deoxyuridine-5′-monophosphate to the antineoplastic drug 5-fluoro-2′-deoxyuridine in human erythrocytes. Proc. Natl. Acad. Sci. USA 85, 3145–3149, 1988.

5. Gasparini, A., Giovine, M., Damonte, G., Tonetti, M., Grandi, T., Mazzei, M., Balbi, A., Silvestro, L., Benatti, U. and De Flora, A. A novel dimeric fluoropyrimidine molecule behaves as a remote precursor of 5-fluoro-2′-deoxyuridine in human erythrocytes. Biochem. Pharmacol. 48, 1121–1128, 1994.
6. Gao, W.Y., Cara, A., Gallo, R. and Lori, F. Low levels of deoxynucleotides in peripheral blood lymphocytes: A strategy to inhibit human immunodeficiency virus type 1 replication. Proc. Natl. Acad. Sci. USA 90, 8925–8928, 1993.
7. Gao, W.Y., Agbaria, R., Driscoll, J.S. and Mitsuya, H. Divergent anti-human immunodeficiency virus activity and anabolic phosphorylation of 2′,3′-dideoxynucleoside analogs in resting and activated human cells. J. Biol. Chem. 269, 12633–12638, 1994.
8. Mitsuya, H., Yarchoan, R. and Broder, S. Molecular targets for AIDS therapy. Science 249, 1533–1544, 1990.
9. Magnani, M., Rossi, L., Brandi, G., Schiavano, G.F., Montroni, M. and Piedimonte, G. Targeting antiretroviral nucleoside analogues in phosphorylated form to macrophages: *in vitro* and *in vivo* studies. Proc. Natl. Acad. Sci. USA 89, 6477–6481, 1992.
10. Magnani, M., Giovine, M., Fraternale, A., Damonte, G., Rossi, L., Scarfi, S., Benatti, U and De Flora, A. Red blood cells as a delivery system for AZT. Drug Delivery 2, 57–61, 1995.
11. Magnani, M., Casabianca, A., Fraternale, A., Brandi, G., Gessani, S., Williams, R., Giovine, M., Damonte, G., De Flora, A. and Benatti, U. Synthesis and targeted delivery of an azidothymidine homodinucleotide conferring protection to macrophages against retroviral infection. Proc. Natl. Acad. Sci. USA 93, 4403–4408, 1996.
12. Perno, C.F., Yarchoan, R., Cooney, D.A., Hartman, N.R.,Gartner, S., Popovic, M., Hao, Z., Gerrard, T.L., Wilson, Y.A., Johns, D.G. and Broder, S. J. Inhibition of human immunodeficiency virus (HIV-1/HTLV-II-IBa-L) replication in fresh and cultured human peripheral blood monocytes/macrophages by azidothymidine and related 2′,3′-dideoxynucleosides. J. Exp. Med. 168, 1111–1125, 1988.
13. Richmann, D.D., Kornbluth, R.S. and Carson, D.A. Failure of dideoxynucleosides to inhibit human immunodeficiency virus replication in cultured human macrophages J. Exp. Med. 166, 1144–1149, 1987
14. Yarchoan, R., Mitsuya, H., Myers, C.E. and Broder, S. Clinical pharmacology of 3′-azido-2′,3′-dideoxythymidine (zidovudine) and related dideoxynucleosides. N. Engl. J. Med. 321, 726–738 1983.
15. Zocchi, E., Tonetti, M., Guida, L., Polvani, C., Benatti, U. and De Flora, A. Encapsulation of doxorubicin in liver-targeted erythrocytes increases the therapeutic index of the drug in a murine metastatic model. Proc. Natl. Acad. Sci. USA 86, 2040–2044, 1989.
16. Zocchi, E., Guida, L., Franco, L., Silvestro, L., Guerrini, M., Benatti, U. and De Flora, A. Free adenosine diphosphate ribose in human erythrocytes: pathways of intraerythrocytic conversion and non enzymic binding to membrane proteins. Biochem. J. 295, 121–130, 1993.

7

ERYTHROCYTE-BASED TARGETED RELEASE TO MACROPHAGES OF AN AZIDOTHYMIDINE HOMODINUCLEOTIDE PREVENTS RETROVIRAL INFECTION

Umberto Benatti,[1] Marco Giovine,[1] Gianluca Damonte,[1] Antonio De Flora,[1] Rosamund Williams,[2] Sandra Gessani,[3] Giorgio Brandi,[4] Anna Casabianca,[5] Alessandra Fraternale,[5] and y Mauro Magnani[5]

[1]Institute of Biochemistry
University of Genoa, Viale Benedetto XV/1
16132 Genoa, Italy
[2]Lepetit Research Center
Gerenzano
21040 Varese, Italy
[3]Laboratory of Virology
Istituto Superiore di Sanità
Viale Regina Elena 299
00161 Romc, Italy
[4]Institute of Hygiene
University of Urbino
Via Saffi 2
61029 Urbino, Italy
[5]Institute of Biochemistry "Giorgio Fornaini"
University of Urbino
Via Saffi 2
61029 Urbino, Italy

1. SUMMARY

Mononuclear phagocytes, representing a known reservoir of HIV-1, feature a poor response to the nucleoside analogues currently used in AIDS therapy. The main reason is a weak phosphorylating activity to start metabolic activation that terminates with the intracellular synthesis of the retroviral reverse transcriptase inhibitors, i.e. the corresponding nucleoside triphosphates. The azidothymidine homodinucleotide ($AZT_{p2}AZT$) recently designed and synthesized in our laboratories proved to be suitable to overcome this limita-

Erythrocytes as Drug Carriers in Medicine, edited by Sprandel and Way
Plenum Press, New York, 1997

tion. $AZT_{p2}AZT$ was encapsulated in erythrocytes where it showed a remarkable stability. This allowed to selectively perturb the membrane of the $AZT_{p2}AZT$-loaded erythrocytes, thereby triggering subsequent opsonization and uptake by macrophage cultures. Macrophages exposed to carrier erythrocytes showed a significant resistance to infection by immunodeficiency viruses. Protection was observed with human, feline and murine macrophages against infection by HIV-1, FIV and LP-BM5 retroviral strains, respectively. These data demonstrate that $AZT_{p2}AZT$-loaded and opsonized erythrocytes represent an efficient "trojan horse" resulting in significant protection of macrophages from retroviral infection.

2. INTRODUCTION

We have previously described the chemical synthesis of a new antiretroviral molecule, azidothymidine dinucleotide ($AZT_{p2}AZT$)[8]. The rationale behind synthesis of this molecule was two-fold. The first was the aim to build up an azidothymidine prodrug ensuring more favourable pharmacokinetic properties as compared to azidothymidine. This expectancy was based on the known occurrence in erythrocytes of a dinucleotide pyrophosphatase and of 5′-nucleotidases, which suggested use of homodinucleotide-loaded red cells as potential slow delivery systems of azidothymidine[7,8]. The second goal was the availability of a prodrug yielding azidothymidine 5′-P in target cells. This is a stringent requirement in mononuclear phagocytes which represent known reservoirs of human immunodeficiency virus (HIV)[3] and which are characterized by a low phosphorylating activity toward antiviral nucleoside analogues including azidothymidine[10].

Since the intraerythrocytic dinucleotide pyrophosphatase activity is weak, most probably as a result of inhibition by ATP[14], we reasoned that $AZT_{p2}AZT$, once encapsulated in erythrocytes, should be stable enough to be targeted to macrophages within reasonably short times. In these cells, pyrophosphatase-catalyzed degradation of $AZT_{p2}AZT$ would yield azidothymidine 5′-P, thus obviating the poor phosphorylating activity that makes resting macrophages rather resistant to the antiviral activity of azidothymidine. On the other hand, erythrophagocytosis is a professional property of macrophages, which has been recently exploited in order to obtain a significant protection of these cells from retroviral infectivity by means of erythrocyte-based targeted delivery of ddCTP[2,6,13].

On these grounds, we developed an "in vitro" system in order to check the effects of selective targeting to macrophages of $AZT_{p2}AZT$, by means of loaded erythrocytes, on susceptibility to subsequent retroviral infection. The results obtained indicated a significant extent of protection of human, feline and murine macrophages from HIV-1, FIV and LP-BM5 immunodeficiency viruses, respectively. These data hold promise on therapeutic applications of this system involving loading of red cells with $AZT_{p2}AZT$ and subsequent membrane perturbation of the carrier erythrocytes to achieve targeting of the carriers to macrophages.

3. EXPERIMENTAL

3.1. Synthesis of $AZT_{p2}AZT$

Synthesis and chemical characterization of $AZT_{p2}AZT$ have been described elsewhere[4,8].

3.2. Analysis of $AZT_{p2}AZT$

Analyses of the parent azidothymidine homodinucleotide and of metabolites thereof were carried out by reverse-phase HPLC, using an ODS-Hypersil C18 column and a linear eluting gradient, as previously described[8].

3.3. Encapsulation of $AZT_{p2}AZT$ in Erythrocytes and Targeting to Macrophages

Encapsulation was carried out according to the standard procedure of hypotonic shock-isotonic resealing and reannealing[1,8], as described. Human, feline and murine red cells were loaded, with minor technical variations among the three species, to reach a final intraerythrocytic concentration of approximately 0.4 μmoles/ml packed cells. For each experiment, loaded, unloaded (i.e., subjected to the encapsulation procedure in the absence of $AZT_{p2}AZT$) and native erythrocyte samples were prepared. The procedure for selective targeting of $AZT_{p2}AZT$-loaded erythrocytes to homologous macrophages has been reported elsewhere[8], as well as the immunological characterization of the opsonized red cells. HPLC analyses of $AZT_{p2}AZT$ were carried out (see above) on perchloric acid extracts of macrophages, neutralized with K_2CO_3 and treated to achieve solid phase extraction of $AZT_{p2}AZT$[1,8]. Following exposure to $AZT_{p2}AZT$-loaded or to unloaded erythrocytes or to 0.1 μM azidothymidine, macrophage cultures were infected with either HIV-$1_{Ba\text{-}L}$, or FIV (Pisa M-2), or LP-BM5, extensively washed and cultured at 37°C and 5% CO_2 for 21, 4 and 4 days, respectively, before assay of infectivity.

3.4. Assays of Antiretroviral Activity or Infected Macrophages

With all virus strains, the antiviral activity was measured in terms of inhibition of proviral DNA formation. For HIV-1 also inhibition of p24 production was evaluated. The experimental details of these assays have been described elsewhere[8].

4. RESULTS

Following encapsulation in human erythrocytes, $AZT_{p2}AZT$ proved to be rather stable. Thus, after 2 hrs incubation of $AZT_{p2}AZT$-loaded erythrocytes in autologous plasma (10% hematocrit), no significant decrease of azidothymidine homodinucleotide was observed and, concomitantly, formation of metabolites thereof was negligible. Such stability was observed within rather wide ranges of encapsulated $AZT_{p2}AZT$, between 0.1 and 4.0

Table 1. p24 production (expressed in ng/ml) in culture supernatants of human macrophages infected with $HIV_{BA\text{-}L}$

Infected	Infected + Unloaded RBC	Infected + AZT dimer	Infected + AZT (20hrs)	Infected + AZT (1 week)
192 ± 8.3	179 ± 7.2	37 ±2.7	182 ± 9	86 ± 3

(from Magnani et al.[8], modified)

μmoles per ml of packed red cells[4]. Comparable patterns were observed in $AZT_{p2}AZT$-loaded feline and murine erythrocytes.

At longer times of incubation, performed under sterile conditions, the encapsulated $AZT_{p2}AZT$ decayed progressively, with a half-life of approximately 70 hrs measured at starting intraerythrocytic levels of 0.15 μmoles per ml of packed red cells[1]. Within this time, the only detectable metabolite was AZT 5′-monophosphate (AZT-MP), while since 24 hrs incubation, the output of azidothymidine from erythrocytes started and progressed linearly with time[1].

This metabolic pattern of azidothymidine formation from encapsulated $AZT_{p2}AZT$ demonstrates the involvement of a dinucleotide pyrophosphatase, eventually followed by a 5′-nucleotidase activity. Such a pyrohosphatase was previously identified and partially purified from human erythrocytes[14]. Its susceptibility to ATP inhibition is likely the mechanism accounting for the observed $AZT_{p2}AZT$ stability within the loaded red cells.

Although delayed azidothymidine formation and release from $AZT_{p2}AZT$-loaded erythrocytes makes these cells potential bioreactors improving pharmacokinetic properties of azidothymidine itself, the marked metabolic stability of $AZT_{p2}AZT$ at short time intervals can be exploited to attempt the relatively fast targeting of these carriers to macrophages. In fact, the procedure of targeting by means of erythrophagocytosis involves times short enough to avoid substantial intraerythrocytic degradation of the red cell-encapsulated $AZT_{p2}AZT$.

Preliminary analysis of the properties of the $AZT_{p2}AZT$-loaded human red cells subjected to membrane perturbation and subsequent opsonization, revealed a significant extent of opsonization (approximately 1,500 IgG molecules/erythrocyte). Average figures of erythrophagocytosis exceeded 1 red cell/macrophage (1.0–1.3). The levels of $AZT_{p2}AZT$ following phagocytosis of erythrocytes containing 0.4 μmol $AZT_{p2}AZT$ per ml were 3 picomol/10^6 human macrophage cells. These levels decreased progressively upon incubation of macrophages, until becoming undetectable after 70 hrs[8]. Since degradation of $AZT_{p2}AZT$ in intact erythrocytes occurs at a consistently slower rate, such decay of azidothymidine homodinucleotide during erythrophagocytosis is clearly occurring within macrophage cells.

The properties of erythrophagocytosis and of subsequent metabolism of $AZT_{p2}AZT$ were quite similar using the feline and the murine homologous systems (not shown).

Although the pathways of $AZT_{p2}AZT$ metabolism in macrophages could not be established, a likely mechanism involves pyrophosphatase-mediated formation of AZT-MP. This compound, if formed in macrophages, might be phosphorylated to yield AZT-DP and AZT-TP, the latter metabolite representing the pharmacologically active molecule responsible for inhibition of viral reverse transcriptase.

In order to check this assumption experimentally, following phagocytosis of $AZT_{p2}AZT$-loaded human, feline and murine erythrocytes, species-specific macrophages were infected with the homologous virus strains, i.e. HIV-1, FIV and LP-BM5, respectively. With the three systems tested, proviral DNA formation was significantly inhibited by the previous exposure of macrophages to the homologous $AZT_{p2}AZT$-loaded, opsonized erythrocytes. The corresponding inhibition figures were 93%-97%, 95% and 71% for the human, feline and murine macrophages, respectively[8].

As shown in Table I, the extent of p24 production was remarkably reduced (down to 19%) in the infected human macrophages exposed to $AZT_{p2}AZT$-loaded, opsonized red cells, as compared to the infected, untreated macrophages. This is a specific effect of the carriers, as unloaded erythrocytes did not reduce p24 production.

Azidothymidine showed some effect, although its presence in the extracellular medium at 0.1 μM was required for the 7 days of the macrophage culture to decrease p24 production significantly. In this case p24 production accounted for 45% of the one observed with the infected and untreated macrophage cells. Exposure of macrophages to 0.1 M azidothymidine over the same time (i.e. 20 hrs) necessary to complete erythrophagocytosis of the $AZT_{p2}AZT$-loaded and opsonized red cells did not determine any significantly decreased p24 production.

5. DISCUSSION

Selective targeting of suitable drugs and prodrugs to macrophages has already been shown to protect these cells from retroviral infection. Protection was demonstrated "in vitro" with HIV-1 and "in vivo" in LP-BM5-infected mice. The erythrocyte-encapsulated antiretroviral drug ddCTP resulted in almost complete inhibition of HIV production and, importantly, this effect was observed in macrophages that had been previously infected[6]. In addition, the "in vivo" study demonstrated reduction of lymphoadenopathy, splenomegaly and hypergammaglobulinemia in C57BL/6 mice that had been previously infected with LP-BM5. Accordingly, the system proved to be highly selective and efficient as it introduced directly in the infected macrophages the reverse transcriptase inhibitor ddCTP[2,6,13].

One of the reasons that suggested the present investigation was the recent demonstration that nucleoside analogs are responsible in the host cells for a serious cytotoxicity which is seemingly afforded by the triphosphorylated nucleoside analogues acting as inhibitors of endogenous enzyme systems[5,9]. Accordingly, an ideal antiviral therapy targeted to the monocyte-macrophage lineage should be based on the continuous occurrence within the infected cells of reasonably low levels of these triphosphorylated nucleoside analogues rather than on the direct delivery of them in a burst fashion.

Azidothymidine homodinucleotide and the targeted system exploiting opsonized erythrocytes seem to fit these pharmacometabolic requirements. Although direct assay of azidothymidine 5′-triphosphate (AZT-TP) was not feasible because of limited sensitivity of the HPLC procedure, this fact by itself demonstrates that the antiretroviral activity observed in our experiments follows the formation of low intracellular levels of pharmacologically active metabolites inhibiting viral reverse transcriptase. This conclusion is strengthened by the fact that $AZT_{p2}AZT$ was a poor "in vitro" inhibitor of recombinant HIV-1 reverse transcriptase, with a K_i above 10 μM. Conversely, the K_i of AZT-TP was 0.05 μM. Therefore, active metabolites of $AZT_{p2}AZT$, likely to be identified, at least in part, with AZT-TP, seem to afford antiviral activity in macrophages[8].

Robbins et al.[12] estimated that in HIV infected patients under effective treatment with azidothymidine, the intracellular concentration of AZT-TP in peripheral blood mononuclear cells ranges from $5 \cdot 10^{-15}$ mol/10^6 cells to $9 \cdot 10^{-14}$ mol/10^6 cells. The actual intracellular concentration of $AZT_{p2}AZT$ in macrophages following phagocytosis of $AZT_{p2}AZT$-loaded, opsonized erythrocytes, was found to be 3.10^{-12} mol/10^6 cells (see Results). This level is approximately tenfold lower than expected on the basis of the observed rate of phagocytosis, i.e. one erythrocyte/macrophage. However, it is still high enough to account for the sustained intracellular formation of AZT-TP levels resulting in effective antiretroviral activity and certainly exceeding those estimated in HIV infected patients receiving standard doses of azidothymidine[12]. In any case, the presumptive AZT-TP intracellular concentrations resulting from the present experimental system are from three to five orders of magnitude lower than those of ddCTP obtained with selective targeting of ddCTP-loaded and opsonized human erythrocytes[5]. This result seems to represent a reasonably safe compromise between the untoward cytotoxic effects of too high intracellular levels of triphosphorylated nucleoside analogues and the too low levels of these pharmacologically active metabolites in macrophages of conventionally treated AIDS patients.

Very recently[11], red blood cells have been shown to be good drug carriers also for a different class of HIV reverse transcriptase inhibitors, i.e. the 9-(2-phosphonylmethoxyethyl)adenine (PMEA). Due to the versatility of the synthesizing procedure developed, other homo- and heterodinucleotides will soon be tested in our laboratories. Preliminary results suggest that this is not only possible but that the therapeutic effects observed are of relevance in a wide number of pathogens endowed in macrophage cells.

6. ACKNOWLEDGMENTS

This study was partially supported by the Italian Ministry of Health, Istituto Superiore di Sanità, Progetto AIDS, and by Gruppo Lepetit S.p.A., Lainate (Milan), Italy.

7. REFERENCES

1. Benatti, U., Giovine, M., Damonte, G., Gasparini, A., Scarfi, S., De Flora, A., Fraternale, A., Rossi, L., Magnani, M. Azidothymidine homodinucleotide- loaded erythrocytes as bioreactors for slow delivery of the antiretroviral drug azidothymidine. Biochem. Biophys. Res. Comm., 220, 20–25, 1996.
2. Fraternale, A., Casabianca, A., Rossi, L., Chiarantini, L., Brandi, G., Aluigi, G., Schiavano, G.F., Magnani, M. Inibition of murine AIDS by combination of AZT and dideoxycytidine 5′-triphosphate. J. Acquir. Immune Defic. Syndr. 12, 164–173, 1996.
3. Gendelman H.E., Meltzer M.S. Mononuclear phagocytes and the human immunodeficiency virus. Curr. Opin. Immunol. 2, 414–419, 1990.
4. Giovine, M., Scarfi, S., Gasparini, A., Millo, E., Damonte, G., De Flora, A., Magnani, M., Fraternale, A., Rossi, L., Williams, R., Benatti, U. Synthesis, characterization and erythrocyte encapsulation of an azidothymidine homodinucleotide behaving as a prodrug of azidothymidine. Biological Carriers in Medicine (U. Sprandel and J.L. Way Eds.) Plenum Press, New York, in press.
5. Lewis, W., Dalakas, M.C., Mitochondrial toxicity of antiviral drugs. Nat. Med. 1, 417–422, 1995
6. Magnani, M., Rossi, L., Brandi, G., Schiavano, G.F., Montroni, M., Piedimonte, G. Targeting antiretroviral nucleoside analogues in phosphorylated form to macrophages: in vitro ed in vivo studies. Proc. Natl. Acad. Sci. USA 89, 6477–6481, 1992.
7. Magnani, M., Giovine, M., Fraternale, A., Damonte, G., Rossi, L., Scarfi, S., Benatti, U., De Flora, A. Red Blood Cells as a Delivery System for AZT. Drug Delivery, 2, 57–61, 1995.
8. Magnani, M., Casabianca, A., Fraternale, A., Brandi G., Gessani, S., Williams, R., Giovine, M., Damonte, G., De Flora, A., Benatti, U. Synthesis and targeted delivery of an azidothymidine homodinucleotide conferring protection to macrophages against retroviral infection. Proc. Natl. Acad. Sci. USA 93, 4403–4408, 1996.
9. Parker, W.B., Cheng, Y.C., Mitochondrial toxicity of antiviral analogs. J. NIH Res. 6, 57–61, 1994.
10. Perno, C.F., Yarchoan, R., Cooney, D.A., Hartman, N.R.,Gartner, S., Popovic, M., Hao, Z., Gerrard, T.L., Wilson, Y.A., Johns, D.G. and Broder, S. J. Inhibition of human immunodeficiency virus (HIV-1/HTLV-II-IBa-L) replication in fresh and cultured human peripheral blood monocytes/macrophages by azidothymidine and related 2′,3′-dideoxynucleosides. J. Exp. Med. 168, 1111–1125, 1988.
11. Perno C.F., Santoro N., Balestra, E., Aquaro S., Lazzarino G., Di Pierro D., Tavazzi B., Balzarini, J., Garaci, E., Grimaldi, S. and Caliò, R. Red blood cells mediated delivery of 9-(2-phosphonylmethoxyethyl)adenine to primary macrophages: efficiency, metabolism and activity against human immunodeficiency virus or herpes simplex virus. Antiv. Res. 33, 153–164, 1997.

12. Robbins, B.L., Rodman, J., McDonald, C., Srinivas, R.V., Flynn, P.M., Fridland, A. Enzymatic assay for measurement of zidovudine triphosphate in peripheral blood mononuclear cells. Antimicrob. Agents Chemother. 38, 115–121, 1994.
13. Rossi, L., Brandi, G:, Fraternale, A., Schiavano, G.F., Chiarantini, L., Magnani, M. Inibition of murine retrovirus induced immunodeficiency disease by dideoxycytidine and dideoxycytidine 5′ triphosphate J. Acquir. Immune Defic. Syndr. 6, 1179–1186, 1993.
14. Zocchi, E., Guida, L., Franco, L., Silvestro, L., Guerrini, M., Benatti, U. and De Flora, A. Free Adenosine diphosphate ribose in human erythrocytes: pathways of intraerythrocytic conversion and non-enzymic binding to membrane proteins. Biochem. J. 295, 121–130, 1993.

THE ENTRAPMENT OF MANNOSE-TERMINATED GLUCOCEREBROSIDASE (ALGLUCERASE) IN HUMAN CARRIER ERYTHROCYTES

Bridget E. Bax,[1] Murray D. Bain,[1] Chandra P. Ward,[2] Anthony H. Fensom,[2] and Ronald A. Chalmers[1]

[1]Paediatric Metabolism Unit
Department of Child Health
St George's Hospital Medical School
London, United Kingdom
[2]SAS Laboratory for Genetic Enzyme Defects
Guy's Hospital
London, United Kingdom

1. INTRODUCTION

The enzyme glucocerebrosidase (β-D-glucosyl-N-acylsphingosine glucohydrolase, EC 3.2.1.45) is responsible for the hydrolytic cleavage of glucose from the glycolipid glucocerebroside within the lysosomes of tissue macrophages. Gaucher's disease is an autosomal recessive, lysosomal storage disorder and is due to a deficiency of glucocerebrosidase. An absence of glucocereobrosidase results in an accumulation of glucocerebroside within the macrophages of the reticulo-endothelial system in the spleen, liver and bone marrow to produce Gaucher cells which are characteristic of this disorder.

Mannose-terminated glucocerebrosidase (Alglucerase) is a licensed pharmaceutical enzyme which provides an enzyme replacement therapy for Gaucher's disease (Sato and Beutler, 1993; Brady, Murray and Barton, 1994). Alglucerase is rapidly cleared from the vascular compartment due to extensive catabolism (half-life of 3.6 to 10.4 minutes); regular infusions are therefore required to maintain therapeutic plasma levels, making therapy both invasive and costly.

In this study we investigated the entrapment of varying concentrations of Alglucerase (molecular weight 59 300) in energy-replete human carrier erythrocytes with the future prospect of using this methodology to target this enzyme in a sustained delivery mechanism to the macrophages of the reticulo-endothelial system, the site of erythrocyte

Erythrocytes as Drug Carriers in Medicine, edited by Sprandel and Way
Plenum Press, New York, 1997

destruction, and thus reduce the dosage and frequency of therapeutic interventions, while enhancing delivery of therapeutic enzyme to the required sites of action.

2. METHODS

2.1. Cell Preparation

Whole blood was collected in heparinized tubes (10 units/ml) from healthy normal volunteers. The erythrocytes were washed twice in cold phosphate buffered saline (PBS) (136.89 mmol/l NaCl, 2.68 mmol/l KCl, 8.10 mmol/l Na_2HPO_4, 1.47 mmol/l KH_2PO_4, pH 7.4) and centrifuged for 10 minutes at 1100g.

2.2. Carrier Erythrocyte Preparation

Energy-replete carrier erythrocytes were prepared using a hypo-osmotic dialysis procedure (Sprandel, Hubbard and Chalmers, 1980; Sprandel, Hubbard and Chalmers, 1981). Seven volumes of washed and packed erythrocytes were mixed with 3 volumes of cold PBS containing varying concentrations of Alglucerase (Genzyme, stock concentration 10 units/ml or 80 units/ml at 25°C). Five ml of this cell suspension were then placed into a 10 ml dialysis bag with a molecular weight cut-off of 12 000 Daltons. After sealing the dialysis bag was placed into a container holding 150 ml hypo-osmotic buffer (5 mmol/l KH_2PO_4, 5 mmol/l K_2HPO_4, pH 7.4) and dialysed at 4°C with rotation at 6 rpm for 90 minutes or (in one experiment) 180 minutes. The lysed erythrocytes were resealed by transferring the dialysis bag to a container holding 150 ml PBS supplemented with 5 mmol/l adenosine, 5 mmol/l glucose and 5 mmol/l $MgCl_2$, pH 7.4 and continuing rotation at 6 rpm for 60 minutes at 37°C. Erythrocytes dialysed in the absence of Alglucerase (unloaded carrier erythrocytes) were prepared to control for Alglucerase assay interference by lysed erythrocytes. The Alglucerase-loaded and unloaded carrier erythrocytes were washed three times in 3 volumes iso-osmotic supplemented PBS, followed by centrifugation at 100g for 15 minutes.

To control for binding of Alglucerase to the outside of the cell membrane during carrier erythrocyte preparation, cells were dialysed with Alglucerase for 90 minutes at 4°C against iso-osmatic PBS (instead of hypo-osmotic buffer), followed by dialysis in supplemented PBS for 60 minutes at 37°C.

2.3. Alglucerase Assay

Entrapped Alglucerase activity was assayed by following the hydrolysis of the synthetic substrate 4-methylumbelliferyl-β-D-glucopyranoside. Diluted and sonicated carrier erythrocytes were incubated with 6.1 mmol/l 4-methylumbelliferyl-β-D-glucopyranoside in 150 mmol/l phosphate/citrate buffer, pH 5.5 and 30.6 mmol/l sodium taurocholate (inhibits non-specific enzyme activity) for 1 hour at 37°C. The reaction was stopped with 500 mmol/l glycine/NaOH buffer, pH 10.3 and the fluorescence of the liberated 4- methylumbelliferone was measured at 448 nm.

3. RESULTS

Figure 1 shows the entrapment of Alglucerase as a function of enzyme concentration in the dialysis tubing using two different pharmaceutically available stock concentrations. Logarithmic scales are used on both axes. Alglucerase entrapment, expressed as a proportion of that initially added to the dialysis bag, was approximately the same for either enzyme concentration. The use of the more concentrated 80 units/ml solution therefore increased Alglucerase entrapment. In one experiment, where a total of 39 units of Alglucerase were added to the dialysis bag, and where the hypo-osmotic dialysis period was increased from 90 minutes to 180 minutes, entrapment was increased by approximately 2-fold (Bax et al.,1996). These results suggest that the entrapment of Alglucerase is limited by its diffusion rate for at least 180 minutes.

No enzyme activity was found to be associated with cells taken through the procedure with dialysis against iso-osmotic PBS demonstrating that Alglucerase does not bind to the outside of the erythrocyte membrane. The carrier erythrocyte-associated Alglucerase is thus entrapped enzyme.

4. CONCLUSIONS

These results show that the combination of the more concentrated pharmaceutical preparation of Alglucerase and extended hypo-osmotic dialysis time enhanced enzyme en-

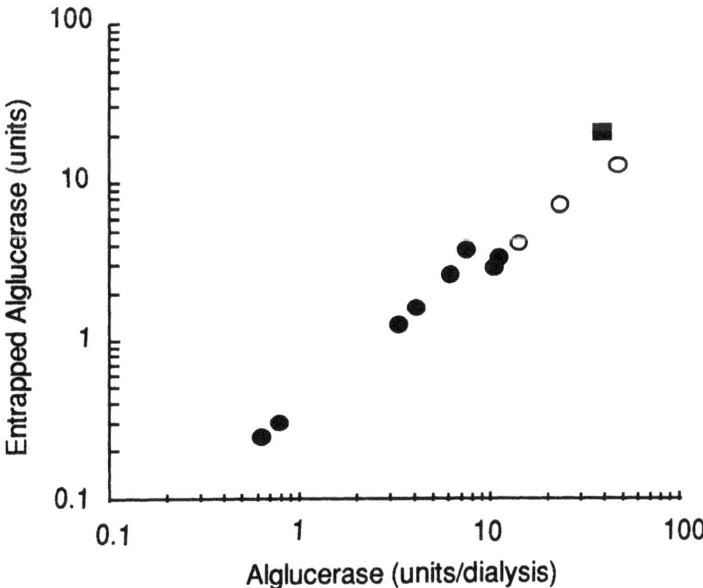

Figure 1. The entrapment of Alglucerase by energy-replete carrier erythrocytes. Each data point represents one dialysis experiment: ● Alglucerase stock concentration 10 units/ml and 90 minutes of hypo-osmotic dialysis; ○ Alglucerase stock concentration 80 units/ml and 90 of minutes hypo-osmotic dialysis; ■ Alglucerase stock concentration 80 units/ml and 180 minutes of hypo-osmotic dialysis. One unit of activity is defined as the amount of enzyme required to convert 1 μmol substrate per minute at 37°C.

trapment. Further studies are in progress to determine the long term effect of entrapped Alglucerase on erythrocyte survival *in vitro*.

5. ACKNOWLEDGMENT

These studies were supported by the Wellcome Trust.

6. REFERENCES

Bax, B.E., Bain, M.D., Ward, C.P., Fensom, A.H. and Chalmers, R.A. The entrapment of mannose-terminated glucocerebrosidase (Alglucerase) in human carrier erythrocytes. Biochem. Soc. Trans. 24: 441S (1996).

Beutler, E. Gaucher's disease. New Engl. J. Med. 25:1354–1360 (1991).

Brady, R.O., Murray, G.J., and Barton N.W. Modifying exogenous glucocerebrosidase for effective replacement therapy in Gaucher disease. J. Inher. Metab. Dis. 17:510–519 (1994).

Chalmers R.A. Comparison and potential of hypo-osmotic and iso-osmotic erythrocyte ghosts and carrier erythrocytes as drug and enzyme carriers. Biblthca. Haemat. 51:15–24 (1985).

Sato, Y. and Beutler, E. Binding, internalization, and degradation of mannose-terminated glucocerebrosidase by macrophages. J. Clin. Invest. 91:1909–1917 (1993).

Sprandel, U., Hubbard, A.R. and Chalmers, R.A. Survival of 'carrier erythrocytes' in dogs. Clin. Sci. 59: 7P (1980).

Sprandel, U., Hubbard, A.R. and Chalmers, R.A. Towards enzyme therapy using carrier erythrocytes. J. Inher. Metab. Dis. 4:99–100 (1981).

9

MACROPHAGE PROTECTION BY NUCLEOSIDE AND NUCLEOTIDE ANALOGUE ADMINISTRATION

L. Rossi,[1] A. Casabianca,[1] A. Fraternale,[1] G. F. Schiavano,[2] G. Brandi,[2] A. Antonelli,[1] and M. Magnani[1]

[1]Institute of Biological Chemistry "Giorgio Fornaini"
[2]Institute of Hygiene
University of Urbino
Italy

1. INTRODUCTION

Cells of the monocyte/macrophage lineage are currently recognized as important targets and reservoirs of human immunodeficiency virus (HIV-1) infection (1, 2). Therefore antiviral strategies, effective in inhibiting virus replication and in preventing transfer of HIV from already infected macrophages to target lymphocytes, must be devised. To date, the most successful anti-HIV therapies are based on compounds that interfere with reverse transcriptase, the viral enzyme required for HIV replication (3). Among these are several dideoxynucleosides, including azidothymidine (AZT), 2′,3′-dideoxycytidine (ddCyd) and 2′,3′-dideoxyinosine (ddI) etc. Each of these compounds is phosphorylated to the active triphosphate form after entring the cell and then acts as a DNA chain terminator and/or a competitor by blocking the incorporation of the respective normal deoxynucleoside-5′-triphosphate (4). The phosphorylation depends on specific cellular kinases whose levels in turn depend on the activation state of the target cells and on the cell types (5). Usually, quiescent cells have low levels of the enzymes responsible for nucleoside analogue phosphorylation, while activation (e.g., mitogen stimulation) results in increased activity levels. Because resting macrophages possess low levels of these kinases, a low efficacy of dideoxynucleoside analogues administration is thought.

However conflicting results (6) have been reported. Furthermore, the ratio of dideoxynucleoside triphosphate analogues to the normal deoxynucleoside triphosphate pool was shown to be important in the drug's activity and macrophages contain low concentrations of deoxynucleosides-5′-triphosphate.

We therefore compared the efficacy of ddCyd and of its active form dideoxycytidine-5′-triphosphate (ddCTP) both in suppressing HIV replication and in inhibiting HIV proviral DNA synthesis in human macrophages. Similar experiments were also performed

Erythrocytes as Drug Carriers in Medicine, edited by Sprandel and Way
Plenum Press, New York, 1997

with the murine immunodeficiency virus (LP-BM5) and the feline immunodeficiency virus (FIV). Because the cell membranes are impermeable to phosphorylated drugs, we have encapsulated ddCTP into autologous erythrocytes and modified the drug-loaded erythrocyte membranes to target these carrier cells to macrophages. The results obtained, show that even ddCyd concentrations higher than those reported to be effective for antiviral activity (6) are less efficient than the direct administration of ddCTP in inhibiting retrovirus replication and proviral DNA integration in macrophages.

2. MATERIALS AND METHODS

2.1. Cell and Virus

Human monocyte-derived macrophages (MDM) were prepared and cultured as in Ref. 7. The purity of isolated macrophages was checked by non-specific esterase staining and was found to be > 95%. Murine macrophages were obtained from the peritoneal cavity of C57BL/6 mice by injection of 5 ml of warm sterile phosphate saline solution (PBS). Abdomens were gently massaged for three minutes and lavage fluids were retrieved by aspiration with a 5 ml syringe. Lavage fluids were centrifuged (1000 g for ten min), cell pellets were washed three times in PBS and then suspended in RPMI-1640 medium containing 10% fetal bovine serum. Peritoneal macrophages (PM) were separated by adherence from non macrophagic cells. Feline MDM cultures were prepared from specific pathogen-free (SPF) cats as described in Ref. 8.

Human macrophages were infected with a preparation of HIV-1 obtained from the supernatant of infected and productive CEM cells. Exposure to the virus was for 24 h at 4 ng p24/10^6 cells. Murine macrophages were infected with LP-BM5 virus, a mixture of murine leukemia viruses (9), prepared as a cell-free supernatant from SC-1 cells as described (10). Exposure to the virus was for 24 h at 3 x 10^6 cpm/10^6 cells of reverse transcriptase (RT). Feline monocyte-derived macrophages were infected with the Pisa-M_2 isolate of FIV propagated in MDM cells as described (11). Exposure to the virus was for 24 h after adding 50–100 µl of virus stock ($TCID_{50}=10^{5.63}$/ml) to each well containing 1 ml of RPMI-1640 medium supplemented with 20% fetal calf serum.

2.2. ddCyd Administration

24 h before exposure to the respective retroviruses human and murine macrophages were cultured in the presence or absence of 1 µM ddCyd while feline macrophage were treated, always with 1.0 µM ddCyd, simultaneously to the infection. The drug was maintained in the medium through out the experiment and the medium was replaced at least once a week. For feline MDM, 0.2 µM ddCyd administration was tested too.

2.3. ddCTP Encapsulation in Erythrocytes

ddCTP was encapsulated in red blood cells (RBC) using a loading procedure consisting in hypotonic dialysis, isotonic resealing and reannealing as described in Ref. 7 for human and murine erythrocytes while as described in Ref. 8 for ddCTP encapsulation in feline erythrocytes. The amount of ddCTP encapsulated in erythrocytes was determined by high-performance liquid chromatography (HPLC) of neutralized $HClO_4$ extracts as described in Ref. 12.

2.4. Targeting of ddCTP-Loaded Erythrocytes to Macrophages

Targeting of ddCTP-loaded RBC to macrophages was achieved by inducing band 3 clustering (band 3 is the major transmembrane protein in the erythrocytes); the clusters, once in serum, are recognized as "non-self" and opsonized by autologous IgG. Targeting procedure is described in detail in Ref. 7.

2.5. ddCTP Administration

ddCTP encapsulated in autologous RBC to a final concentration of 1 μmol/ml was added to the human and murine macrophage cultures 24 h before infection while to feline macrophages simultaneously to the infection at a ratio of 100 RBC per macrophage. Non ingested erythrocytes were removed with the free virions 24 h after infection. In murine macrophages the condition 0.2 μmol ddCTP/ml RBC was tested too while in feline macrophage the efficacy of 0.4 μmol ddCTP/ml RBC was evaluated. In all the experiments, erythrocytes processed as for the encapsulation of ddCTP but without any drug addition (unloaded, UL) were used as controls.

2.6. Assays of Antiviral Activity

Inhibition of HIV-1 and FIV production was determined by measurement of released RT activity in the culture supernatant using poly (A) oligo $(dT)_{12-18}$ as template primer with 5 mM Mg^{2+} and $[^3H]$-thymidine-5′-triphosphate (13). As murine macrophages produce very small amounts of the LP-BM5 virus, values of RT cannot be accurately determined. The efficacy of drug administration in inhibiting LP-BM5 production in murine macrophages was therefore evaluated by the analyses of Pr-60^{gag} expression. To this purpose an immunocytochemistry method was used (14).

2.7. Determination of HIV and LP-BM5 proviral DNA content

Total cellular DNA extraction, primers and probes used and PCR analyses were performed as described in Ref. 15.

3. RESULTS

3.1. Suppression of HIV Replication in Macrophages

Human monocyte-derived macrophages were cultured for 10 days before receiving 1 μM ddCyd or red blood cells loaded with ddCTP to a final concentration of 1 μmol/ml. 24 hours later, the cells were infected for 24 h with HIV-LAI 4 ng p24/10^6 macrophages and then six times washed with fresh medium. The cellular cultures were kept at 37°C, 5% CO_2 and the medium changed every week. For the cells treated with ddCyd, the drug was present in the medium through out the experiment. As shown in Fig. 1, ddCTP administered to macrophages by carrier erythrocytes was more efficient than ddCyd in inhibiting retrovirus replication in human macrophages.

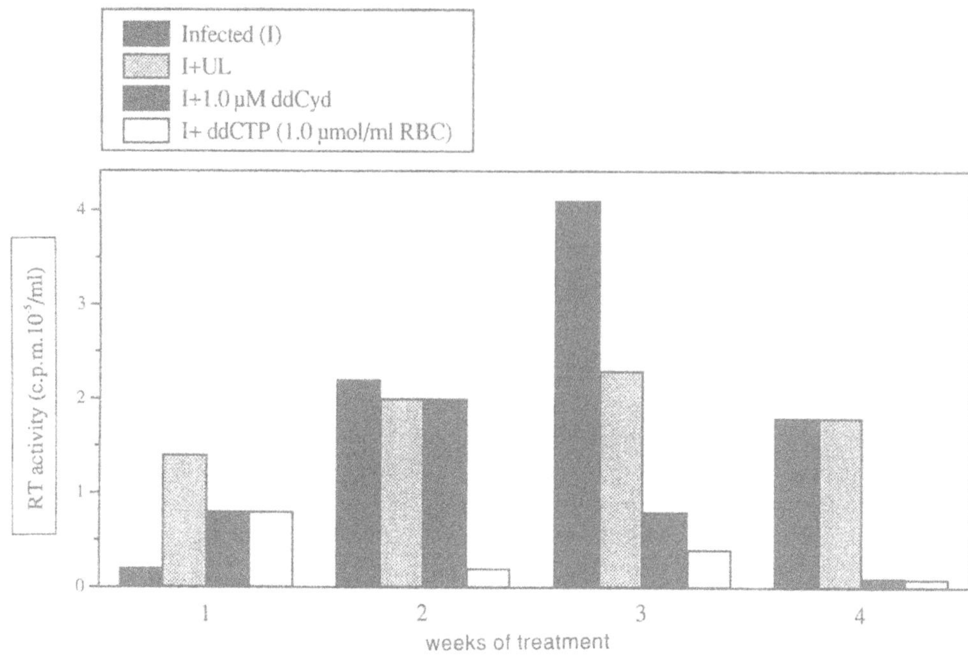

Figure 1. Suppression of virus replication in human macrophages by ddCyd or ddCTP-loaded erythrocytes. Human monocyte-derived macrophages were cultured and treated as described under "Materials and Methods" section. All values are means of at least three different experiments and agree within 10%.

3.2. Proviral HIV-1 in Macrophages

4 weeks after infection, the HIV-1 proviral DNA content in human macrophages receiving ddCyd or ddCTP-loaded RBC was evaluated. The results reported in tab.1 show an high efficacy (93%) of loaded RBC in inhibiting the synthesis and the integration of proviral DNA in the host genome. The treatment with ddCyd resulted in a partial inhibition of HIV-1 infectivity with values almost similar to those obtained with the UL RBC administration.

Table 1. Inhibition of HIV-1 proviral DNA integration in human macrophages treated with ddCyd or ddCTP-loaded RBC

Drug added	% inhibition of HIV-1 proviral DNA content
None	0
Unloaded	61 ± 3
ddCyd (1 µM)	77 ± 4
ddCTP (1.0 µmol/ml RBC)	93 ± 3

Proviral DNA content was evaluated respect to HIV-1 infected and not treated human macrophages. The values were obtained by laser scan densitometry of the autoradiographic films and are mean ± S.D. of three experiments.

3.3. Suppression of LP-BM5 Replication in Macrophages

Murine macrophages collected from the peritoneal cavity of C57BL/6 mice were "in vitro" infected by the LP-BM5 retrovirus complex. Also if no RT activity was found in the medium during three weeks of culture, the expression of Pr-60^{gag} on cellular surface was revealed. Therefore, the efficacy of drug treatment on LP-BM5 replication was evaluated following the virus expression by Pr-60^{gag} immunostaining. As shown in Fig. 2, already after two weeks of culture the ddCTP-loaded RBC administration resulted in a reduced number of cells positive for Pr-60^{gag} expression respect to ddCyd treatment. However the antibody used does not discriminate between Pr-60^{gag} products of ecotropic and defective viruses. These results should be therefore interpretate with caution.

3.4. LP-BM5 proviral DNA in macrophages

LP-BM5 infected macrophages were cultured for three weeks in presence of 1.0μM ddCyd and two different concentrations (0.2 and 1.0 μM). LP-BM5 proviral DNA load was evaluated by PCR analyses and the results are as reported in Tab. 2.

3.5. Suppression of FIV Replication in Macrophages

Feline monocyte-derived macrophages were obtained and infected as decribed under "Materials and Methods" section. ddCyd and ddCTP treatments began simultaneously to the infection. The efficacy of ddCTP-loaded erythrocytes in inhibiting FIV replication in macrophages was evaluated after 2 weeks in culture and compared with that of ddCyd. As

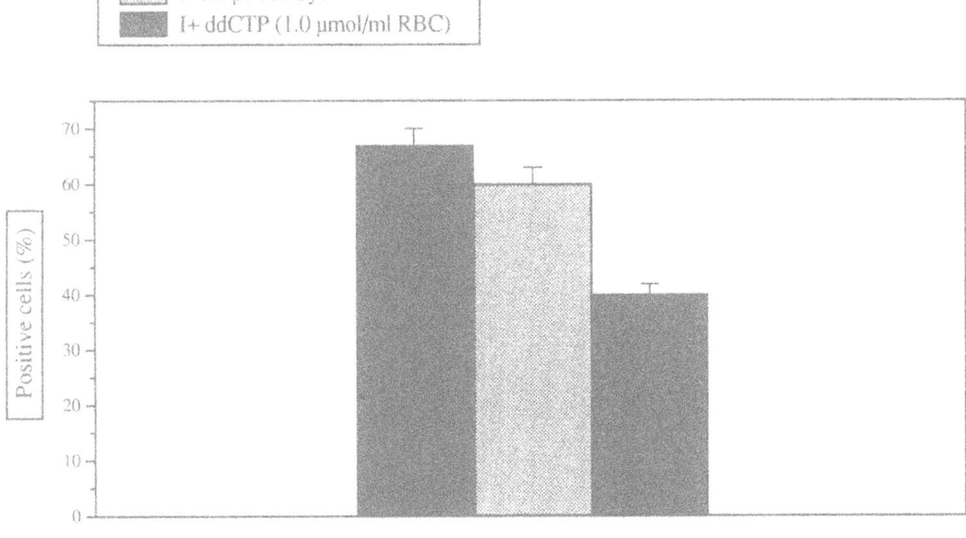

Figure 2. Counting of Pr-60^{gag} positive cells after ddCyd or ddCTP administration to infected murine macrophages. Murine peritoneal macrophages were cultured and treated as described under "Materials and Methods" section. The values are mean ± SD of three different experiments with counts of least 50 cells/sample.

Table 2. Inhibition of LP-BM5 DNA integration in murine macrophages treated with ddCyd or ddCTP-loaded RBC

Drug added	% inhibition of LP-BM5 proviral DNA content
None	0
Unloaded RBC	10 ± 2
ddCyd (1 μM)	56 ± 4
ddCTP (0.2 μmol/ml RBC)	90 ± 2
ddCTP (1.0 μmol/ml RBC)	99 ± 2.5

Proviral DNA content was evaluated respect to the LP-BM5 infected and not treated murine macrophages. The values were obtained by laser scan densitometry of the autoradiographic films and are mean ± S.D. of three experiments.

shown in Fig. 3, two different concentrations of both drugs were tested. The results obtained showed that therapeutic ddCyd concentration (0.2 μM) is without efficacy in protecting macrophagic compartment while 50% of inhibition of viral replication was found with the higher (1.0 μM) ddCyd concentration. Better results were obtaining by administration of 1.0 μmoles ddCTP/ml RBC where 98% of inhibition of FIV replication was found. Differently, only 30% of inhibition was achieved after administration of 0.4 μmol ddCTP/ml RBC to infected macrophage cultures.

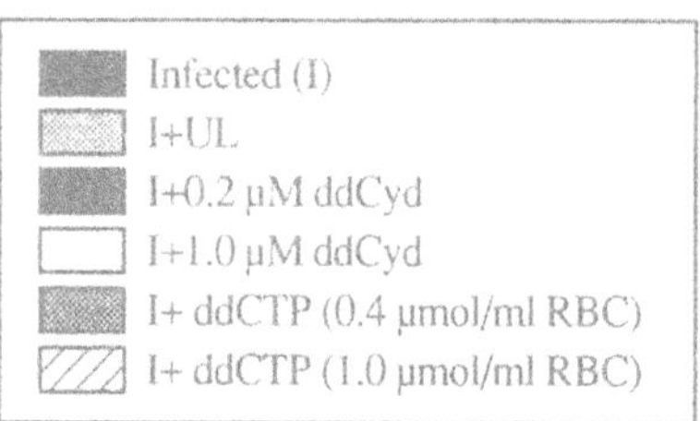

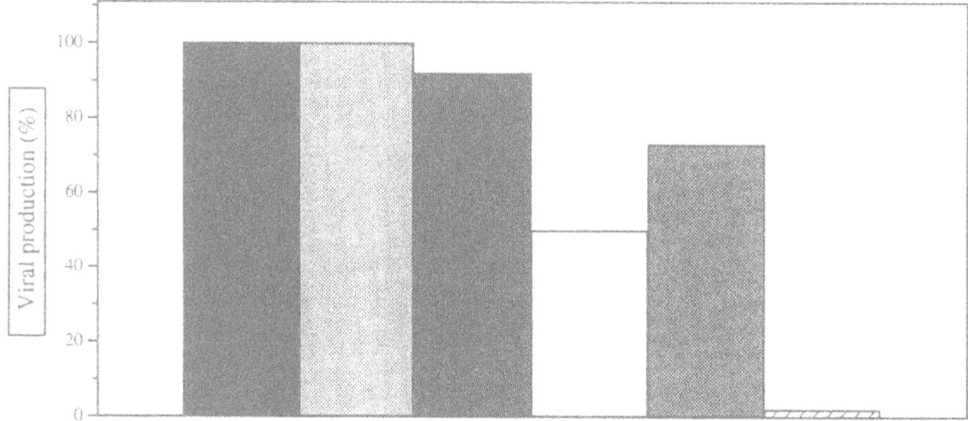

Figure 3. Inhibition of FIV replication in monocyte-derived macrophages by ddCyd or ddCTP-loaded erythrocytes. Feline monocyte-derived macrophages were prepared as described in Ref. 8. One hundred percent viral production was determined after two weeks in culture and corresponding to 210,000 cpm of RT. All values are mean of three determinations and agree within 5%.

4. CONCLUSIONS

HIV-1 resides at low rates of replication in macrophages without producing classic cytopathic effects. Since in this state the virus can infect T lymphocytes, the macrophage acts as a reservoir and propagator of virions throughout the immune system (16). Unfortunately well-differentiated macrophages posses low abilities to phosphorylate (and consequently activate) the most common reverse transcriptase inhibitors of the nucleoside analogue family compared to T cells (17). However 2′,3′-dideoxycytidine, a nucleoside analogue phosphorylated by deoxycytidine kinase, has been reported to be effective in inhibiting HIV-1 replication in macrophages (6). It is not known whether this inhibition is a result of the action of 2′,3′-dideoxycytidine-5′-triphosphate (ddCTP) on HIV reverse transcriptase or of the depletion caused by dideoxycytidine (ddCyd) of the cellular concentration of deoxycytidine-5′-triphosphate (dCTP) needed for synthesis of HIV-1 DNA (18). In this case, low levels of dCTP alone should be sufficient to inhibit the activity of reverse transcriptase and reduce HIV-1 replication without any ddCTP implication. In an attempt to investigate the real role of ddCyd, we tested its ability in inhibiting HIV-1 replication in macrophages at concentrations 100 times those reported (6) to be effective for antiviral activity and compared the results with those obtained by administration of ddCTP using autologous RBC as a drug-delivery system. This last approach overcomes the low ability of the cell to phosphorylate ddCyd and provides direct evidence for the role of ddCTP as an RT inhibitor. The results obtained using 1 μM ddCyd confirm the antiviral activity of the drug showing a partial inhibition both of viral replication (50% inhibition of RT at peak) and of HIV-1 DNA integration (77% of inhibition). However, better results were obtained by administering ddCTP-loaded RBC. We have performed similar experiments on feline macrophages too since FIV and HIV are both lentiviruses and their RT are both sensitive to inhibition by dideoxynucleoside analogues (19). The results obtained were very similar to those achieved in human macrophages confirming that ddCTP-loaded erythrocytes were more efficient than 1 μM ddCyd in inhibiting FIV replication. Furthermore, since murine cells are less sensitive to ddCyd as a result of limited phosphorylation (20), we thought that LP-BM5 infected macrophages could represent an ideal cellular model to evaluate the role of nucleoside phosphorylation in the inhibition of retrovirus infectivity. Analyses of Pr-60^{gag} expression and LP-BM5 proviral DNA synthesis showed that ddCTP-loaded erythrocytes were again more efficient than ddCyd in inhibiting the viral replication. Thus, ddCyd was found to inhibit partially HIV-1, FIV and LP-BM5 replication in macrophages. Concentrations of ddCyd higher than 1 μM were not tested because they are toxic in vivo and in vitro (21) also if this toxicity did not involve macrophages. Phagocytosis of latex beads, production of superoxide anions upon stimulation with latex and phorbol esters and spontaneous production of TNF-α and IL-1β by macrophages treated with 1.0 μM ddCyd or 1 mM ddCTP-loaded RBC, were similar to those of macrophages receiving no drug treatment. However, in human macrophages subjected for six weeks to therapeutic dose (0.1 μM) of ddCyd, an increasing depletion of mitochondrial DNA responsible of a delayed toxicity was observed (data not shown). Since ddCTP concentration in macrophages receiving 1 mM ddCTP-loaded RBC is undetectable a week later, no delayed toxicity is expected. Therefore, ddCTP-loaded erythrocytes have at least two potential advantages over ddCyd: they overcome the limitations caused by the reduced phosphorylation in macrophages and can be used at a wider range of concentrations than ddCyd since the drug is delivered only to macrophages where its toxicity is negligible.

In conclusion, from the available date, is not possible to determine the reason for the limited efficacy of ddCyd, however, it is evident that the limited anabolic phosphorylation of this drug in macrophages plays a major role. Despite the fact that ddCyd reduces the cellular concentrations of ddCTP and/or inhibits HIV-1 RT as ddCTP, it is not efficient enough to abrogate a productive HIV-1 infection in macrophages.

ACKNOWLEDGMENTS

This work was supported by Ministero della Sanità, Istituto Superiore di Sanità, Progetto AIDS 1996. We grateful thank Prof. M. Bendinelli, University of Pisa, Italy, for providing FIV and helpful discussion.

REFERENCES

1. Levy, J.A., Shimabukuro, J., McHugh, T., Casavant, C., Stites, D., Oshiro, L. (1985). AIDS associated retroviruses (ARV) can productively infected other cells besides human T helper cells. Virology 147, 441–447.
2. Ho, D.D., Rota, T.R., Hirsch, M.S. (1986). Infection of monocyte/macrophages by human T lymphocyte virus type III. J. Clin. Invest. 77, 1712–1715.
3. Hirsch, M.S. and D'Aquila, R.T. (1993). Therapy for human immunodeficiency virus infection. N. Engl. J. Med. 328, 1686–1695.
4. De Clerq, E. (1991). Basic approaches to antiretroviral treatment. J. AIDS 4, 207–218.
5. Gao, W. Agbaria, R., Driscoll, J.S. and Mitsuya, H. (1994). Divergent anti-human immunodeficiency virus activity and anabolic phosphorylation of 2′,3′-dideoxynucleoside analogs in resting and activated human cells. J. Biol. Chem. 269, 12633–12638.
6. Perno, C., Yarchoan, R., Cooney, D.A., Hartman, N.R., Gartner, S., Popovic, M., Hao, Z., Garrard, T.L., Wilson, Y.A., Johns, D.G. and Broder, S. (1988). Inhibition of human immunodeficiency virus (HIV-1/HTLV-III BA-L) replication in fresh and cultured human peripheral blood monocyte/macrophages by azidothymidine and related 2′,3′-dideoxynucleosides. J. Exp. Med. 168, 1111–1125.
7. Magnani, M., Rossi, L., Brandi G., Schiavano, G.F., Montroni, M. and Piedimonte, G. (1992). Targeting antiretroviral nucleoside analogues in phosphorylated form to macrophages: in vitro and in vivo studies. Proc. Natl. Acad. Sci. U.S.A. 89, 6477–6481.
8. Magnani, M., Rossi, L., Fraternale, A., Silvotti, L., Quintavalla, F., Piedimonte, G., Matteucci, D., Baldinotti, F. and Bendinelli, M. (1994). Feline immunodeficiency virus infection of macrophages: in vitro and in vivo inhibition by dideoxycytidine-5′-triphosphate-loaded erythrocytes. AIDS Res. Hum. Retrovirus 10(9), 1179–1186.
9. Chattopadhyay, S.K., Sengupta, D.N., Fredrickson, T.N., Morse III, H.C. and Hartley, J.L. (1991). Characteristic and contributions of defective, ecotropic and mink cell focus-inducing viruses involved in a retrovirus induced immunodeficiency syndrome of mice. J. Virol. 65, 4232–4241.
10. Mosier, D.E., Yetter, R.A. and Morse III, H.C. (1987). Functional T lymphocytes are required for a murine retrovirus induced immunodeficiency disease (MAIDS). J. Exp. Med. 165, 1737–1742.
11. Matteucci, D., Baldinotti, F., Mazzetti, P., Pistello, M., Bandecchi, P., Ghilarducci, R., Poli, A., Tazzini, F. and Bendinelli, M. (1993). Detection of feline immunodeficiency virus in saliva and plasma by cultivation and polymerase chain reaction. J. Clin. Microbiol. 31, 494–501.
12. Brandi, G., Rossi, L., Schiavano, G.F., Salvaggio, L., Albano, A. and Magnani, M. (1991). In vitro toxicity and metabolism of 2′,3′-dideoxycytidine, an inhibitor of human immunodeficiency virus infectivity. Chem. Biol. Interactions 79, 53–64.
13. Barrè-Sinoussi, F., Chermann, J.C., Rey, F., Nugeyre, M.T., Chamaret, S., Gruest, J., Dauget, C., Axler-Blin, C., Vezinet, F., Ronzioux, C., Rozenbaum, W. and Montagnier, L. (1983). Isolation of a T-lymphotropic retrovirus from a patient at risk for acquired immune deficiency syndrome (AIDS). Science 220: 868–871.

14. Rossi, L., Brandi, G., Fraternale, A., Schiavano, G.F., Chiarantini, L. and Magnani, M. (1993). Inhibition of murine retrovirus-induced immunodeficiency disease by dideoxycytidine and dideoxycytidine 5′-triphosphate. J. Acq. Imm. Def. Synd. 6, 1179–1186.
15. Magnani, M., Casabianca, A., Rossi, L., Fraternale, A., Brandi, G., Silvotti, L. and Piedimonte, G. (1995). Inhibition of HIV-1 and LP-BM5 replication in macrophages by dideoxycytidine and dideoxycytidine 5′-triphosphate. Antiv. Chem. & Chemother. 6, 312–319.
16. Meltzer, M.S., Skillman, D.R., Gomatos, P.J., Kalter, D.C. and Gendelman, H.E. (1990). Role of mononuclear phagocytes in the pathogenesis of human immunodeficiency virus infection. Ann. Rev. Immunol. 8, 169–194.
17. Richman, D.D., Kombluth, R.S. and Carson, D.A. (1987). Failure of dideoxynucleosides to inhibit human immunodeficiency virus replication in cultured human macrophages. J. Exp. Med. 166, 1144–1149.
18. Gao, W., Cara, A., Gallo, R. and Lori, F. (1993). Low levels of deoxynucleotides in peripheral blood lymphocytes: a strategy to inhibit human immunodeficiency virus type 1 replication. Proc. Natl. Acad. Sci. U.S.A. 90, 8925–8928.
19. North, T.W., Cronn, R.C., Remington, K.M. and Tandberg, R.T. (1990). Direct comparison of inhibitor sensitivities of reverse transcriptases from feline and human immunodeficiency viruses. Antimicrob. Agents Chemother. 34, 1505–1507.
20. Rossi, L., Brandi, G., Schiavano, G.F., Chiarantini, L., Albano, A. and Magnani, M. (1992). In vitro and in vivo toxicity of 2′,3′-dideoxycytidine in mice. Chem. Biol. Interactions 85, 255–263.
21. Chen, C.H. and Cheng, Y.C. (1989), Delayed cytotoxicity and selective loss of mitochondrial DNA in cells treated with the anti-human immunodeficiency virus compound 2′,3′-dideoxycytidine. J. Biol. Chem. 264, 11934–11937.

10

INHIBITION OF MURINE AIDS BY COMBINATION OF AZT AND DDCTP-LOADED ERYTHROCYTES

A. Fraternale,[1] A. Casabianca,[1] L. Rossi,[1] L. Chiarantini,[1] G. Brandi,[2] G. Aluigi,[1] G. F. Schiavano,[2] and M. Magnani[1]

[1]Institute of Biological Chemistry "Giorgio Fornaini"
[2]Institute of Hygiene
University of Urbino
Italy

1. INTRODUCTION

The human acquired immunodeficiency syndrome (AIDS) is a complex disease induced by the human immunodeficiency virus (1, 2). The development of effective therapies for AIDS has been limited by the lack of animal models that exactly mimic events in human disease. Murine AIDS (MAIDS) is a disease that shares many similarities with human AIDS such as splenomegaly, hypergammaglobulinemia, lymphoadenopathy, T- and B-lymphocyte dysfunctions and profound immunodeficiency (3–5). Since many features of this syndrome are common to those defined in human AIDS, MAIDS serve as a useful experimental model for understanding the pathogenesis of AIDS as well as searching for anti-HIV drugs. In our laboratory this animal model has been used to evaluate the efficacy and toxicity of drugs belonging to the nucleoside analogue family (6, 7), known to be potent in vitro and in vivo inhibitors of HIV-1 replication. Unfortunately, the efficacy of drugs so far used in monotherapy is of limited duration while a number of preliminary studies have already shown that combination therapy is more effective than monotherapy (8, 9). Combination therapy may provide additive or synergistic effect of combined drugs, decreased toxicity and delay of viral resistance. Furthermore, treatment can include drugs acting at different levels of HIV replication or protecting different cell types (i.e. lymphocytes and macrophages). Monocyte/macrophages are important target cells for the human immunodeficiency virus type 1 (HIV-1) (10, 11). They may be chronic recervoirs of HIV-1 and probably play an important role in the pathogenesis of AIDS-related complications such as dementia. Unfortunately, nucleoside analogues are not very effective in protecting macrophages from HIV-1 infection because of the low phosphorylating activities of these cells. In fact, the phosphorylation reactions crucial to the activation of the nucleoside analogues are catalysed by host cell kinases: to overcome this problem we encapsulated the

Erythrocytes as Drug Carriers in Medicine, edited by Sprandel and Way
Plenum Press, New York, 1997

active form of 2′,3′-dideoxycytidine (ddCTP) into erythrocytes. Subsequently, the encapsulated antiviral drug was targeted to cells of the monocyte-macrophage (M/M) lineage by treatments that increase the binding of autologous immunoglobulins on the RBC surface. In this way the content of the erythrocyte (ddCTP) becomes available in the monocytic cells where we have shown it is able to inhibit viral infectivity and replication in murine macrophages in vitro (12) and to reduce the typical signs of MAIDS in vivo (13).

On the other hand, it was already reported that AZT at the concentration of 0.25 mg/ml is able to protect mice infected with LP-BM5 MuLV from severe immunodeficiency (14, 15). The combination of ddCTP encapsulated in red blood cells to protect macrophages and AZT to protect lymphocytes could be more effective than a single drug. In this study we evaluated the efficacy of this two-drug treatment in the murine retrovirus-induced immunodeficiency model of AIDS (MAIDS).

2. METHODS

LP-BM5 was kindly provided by Robert Yetter (Veterans Administration Hospital, Baltimore, MD, U.S.A.) and was maintained in a persistently infected SC-1 cell line as described (16). C57BL/6 female mice (purchased from Nossan, Milan, Italy) were used at 5 weeks of age and were infected by a single i.p. injection of 0.1 ml of the virus stock containing 6 x 10^6 cpm of reverse transcriptase. Mice were housed at 22 ± 1°C with 12 h light/dark cycle, 60 ± 5% humidity, and 12 air changes/h.

2.1. AZT

AZT (Sigma) was administered ad libitum in the drinking water at a concentration of 250 mg/l for the duration of the experiment beginning 24 h after infection. AZT was stable in the drinking water at room temperature and was changed every 3 days. The concentration of AZT in drinking water was determined by high-performance liquid chromatography (HPLC) and found to be 0.248 ±0.0014 mg/ml. The plasma concentration of AZT in animals receiving the highest drug concentration was 1.25 ± 0.05 μM. This value was obtained by HPLC on pooled blood samples from three animals bled in the morning and from three bled in the afternoon.

2.2. ddCTP Encapsulation in Erythrocytes

ddCTP was encapsulated in murine erythrocytes as described (13). Targeting of ddCTP-loaded erythrocytes to macrophages was achieved by inducing band 3 clustering (band 3 is the major transmembrane protein in the erythrocyte). These clusters, once in serum, are recognized and opsonized by autologous IgG and complement, thus promoting phagocytosis of the drug-loaded erythrocytes (13). ddCTP-loaded erythrocytes contain 1.7 ± 0.6 μmoles ddCTP/ml erythrocytes and bind 3,000 to 4,500 molecules of IgG/erythrocyte. ddCTP-loaded erythrocytes were administered intraperitoneally in an amount of 200 μl at a hematocrit of 7%. The first administration was 24 h after incubation.

2.3. Preparation of Cellular DNA

Total cellular DNA was isolated from lymph nodes and spleen by lysis with 8 M urea, 0.3 M NaCl and 10 mM Tris-HCl, pH 7.5, for 60 min at 37°C. Extraction was with phenol-chloroform-isoamyl alcohol (25:24:1) and then with chloroform-isoamyl alcohol (24:1). The DNAs were precipitated with ethanol and stored at -20°C until use in the PCR reaction. DNA to be used in PCR amplifications was quantified with Pico Green quantitation reagent from Molecular Probes, Inc. (Eugene, OR, U.S.A.)

2.4. Probes

Probe D30, which was derived from the 137-bp *SmaI-XhoI p12 gag* fragment of the defective virus genome (DU5H) (17) was kindly provided by P. Jolicoeur (Montreal, Canada).

The probe glucose-6-phosphate dehydrogenase (G6PD) represented the 203-bp of the murine genome. G6PD gene probe was obtained in our laboratory by PCR using the following oligonucleotide primers: 5′primer, 5′-TGTTCTTCAACCCCGAGGAGT-3′ (sense) and 3′primer, 5′-AAGACGTCCAGGATGAGGTGATC-3′ (antisense) (18).

2.5. PCR Analyses of LP-BM5 proviral DNA

The following oligonucleotide primers were used for the amplification of defective virus genome (BM5d): 5′primer, 5′-AACCTTCCTCCTCTGCCA-3′ (sense) corresponding to nucleotides 1456–1473 in the viral sequence and 3′primer, 5′-ACCACCTCTCGGGTTTC-3′ (antisense) corresponding to nucleotides 1579–1596 of the BM5d genome (19). A second pair of oligonucleotide primers was used for amplification of 203-bp of the mouse G6PD gene. This amplification served as an internal control (endogenous standard) for evaluation of relative BM5d integration in the mouse genome.

The nucleotide primers for this amplification were as follows: 5′primer, 5′-TGTTCTTCAACCCCGAGGAGT-3′ (sense) and 3′primer, 5′-AAGACGTCCAGGATGAGGTGATC-3′ (antisense).

PCR was performed in a Perkin-Elmer thermocycler in a 25 μl final volume containing 1 μg of genomic DNA, 50 mM KCl, 10 mM Tris-HCl, pH 8.3, 1 mM $MgCl_2$, 0.005% NP-40, 0.001% gelatin, 150 μM each of the four deoxyribonucleoside triphosphates, 20 pmol of each primer and 2.5 U of Replitherm DNA polymerase (Epicentre, Madison, Wisconsin). The reaction mixtures were subjected to 37 cycles of denaturation at 95°C for 30 s, annealling at 58°C for 30 s, and extension at 72°C for 30 s followed by final extension at 72°C for 10 min. The PCR products were analysed by electrophoresis on 2.5% agarose gel, transferred onto nylon membrane and hybridized with either the ^{32}P-labelled D30 or G6PD probe. Labelling of the DNA probes was achieved using the random primer DNA-labelling kit from Bio-Rad (Richmond, CA, U.S.A.).

2.6. Serum Immunoglobulin Determination

Serum IgG levels were determined using an ELISA technique. Briefly, polyvinylchloride microtitre plates (Sterilin, Hounslow, UK) were coated with serial dilutions of murine serum in 50 mM sodium borate, pH 8.5, and incubated for 48 h at 4°C. The plates were washed four times with 0.05% Tween 20 in phosphate-buffered saline (TPBS) and blocked with 1.2% BSA in TPBS for 30 min at room temperature. After two washings in TPBS, 100 μl of goat anti-mouse IgG horseradish peroxidase (HRP)-conjugate (Bio-Rad, Richmond, CA), diluted 1:3000 in 0.2% BSA in TPBS, was added. After incubation for 3 h at room temperature, the plates were washed four times in TPBS and serum IgG was determined using a colour development solution containing 2.2 mM o-phenylenediamine.

Absorbance was measured at 492 nm on Model 2550 EIA READER (Bio-Rad). Absolute serum IgG concentrations were obtained using known concentrations of standard mouse IgG.

3. RESULTS

The LP-BM5 murine leukemia virus (MuLV) causes a syndrome, termed murine AIDS (MAIDS) characterized by early onset of lymphoadenopathy, splenomegaly, hypergammaglobulinemia and deficiencies of both B and T cell responses to polyclonal and antigenic stimuli. Also, a major reservoir and primary site of infection is in the monocyte-macrophage, similar to the case in human AIDS. To protect macrophages we encapsulated ddCTP into erythrocytes that have been modified to increase their recognition by macrophages. We had already demonstrated that this system is able to inhibit LP-BM5 infectivity and expression in murine macrophages in vitro (12) and to delay murine AIDS in LP-BM5-infected mice (13).

We administered ddCTP-loaded erythrocytes to protect macrophages in combination with AZT to protect lymphocytes. ddCTP was encapsulated in murine erythrocytes by a procedure of hypotonic dialysis and isotonic resealing as described in "Methods". Following this procedure ddCTP was encapsulated in murine red blood cells at a final concentration of about 1.7 mM. The first administration was 24 h after infection and then once every 10 days. AZT was administered in drinking water at the concentration of 250 mg/l. Two groups of animals served as controls: one group of 10 mice was not infected, the other one was infected and treated with "unloaded" erythrocytes that are erythrocytes treated as in the procedure of ddCTP encapsulation but without added drug. After 7 and 13 weeks of treatment 5 animals per group were sacrified and splenomegaly, lymphoadenopathy and hypergammaglobulinemia evaluated. In Tab. 1 it is shown the reduction of splenomegaly and lymphoadenopathy of animals treated with AZT and erythrocytes ddCTP-loaded. This reduction is more pronounced than that obtained by AZT or ddCTP alone (not shown).

Results obtained by the evaluation of hypergammaglobulinemia show that the combination of AZT and erythrocytes ddCTP-loaded is more effective than single drugs in inhibiting the levels of circulating IgG at 7 weeks but not at 13 weeks (Tab. 2).

We analysed the BM5d proviral DNA content of spleen and lymph nodes of animals treated with both drugs (Fig. 1). The drug combination provided a reduction of proviral DNA of 72.4±9% in the spleen and 82.8±8% in lymph nodes (mean ± S.D. of 5 animals). Finally evaluation of several haematological parameters did not show any particular toxicity in mice receiving both treatments (Tab. 3).

Table 1. Inhibition of MAIDS by the combination of AZT and ddCTP-loaded erythrocytes

	Body weight (g)		Spleen weight (g)		Lymphnode weight (g)	
Mice	7 weeks	13 weeks	7 weeks	13 weeks	7 weeks	13 weeks
Controls	18.2±0.5	21.2±0.4	0.08±0.02	0.09±0.01	0.05±0.02	0.03±0.01
Infected (I)+ "unloaded" RBC	18.9±0.6	25.2±1.2	0.27±0.02	1.22±0.42	0.35±0.02	3.78±0.61
I+AZT+ddCTP	19.3±2.0	21.5±1.6	0.14±0.05	0.27±0.16	0.10±0.06	0.29±0.12

Values are means ± S.D. of 5 animals.

Table 2. Percentage of inhibition of hypergammaglobulinemia in mice infected with LP-BM5 and treated with AZT and erythrocytes ddCTP-loaded

	7 weeks	13 weeks
I+AZT	60%	50%
I+ddCTP	45%	25%
I+AZT+ddCTP	82%	50%

The percentage of inhibition has been calculated respect to infected and not treated animals.

4. DISCUSSION

It is known that AZT and other available nucleosides such as ddC, ddI etc are effective in inhibiting HIV-1 production in vitro and delaying disease progression in patients. Unfortunately long-term antiviral therapy has been complicated by the emergence of resistant HIV-1 strains, toxic effects and low efficacy in some cells such as macrophages. Combination therapy of AIDS has several potential advantages. One is the potential for reducing toxicity combining drugs with different toxicity profiles. Another reason for combining various drugs is the potential for drug synergy. In addition, different drugs may achieve more effective antiviral activity when properly combined; for example drugs acting at different levels of HIV replication or at different cells can be combined. In this study we evaluated the efficacy of intraperitoneal administration of erythrocytes ddCTP-loaded combined with the administration of AZT in drinking water. In fact we had previously demonstrated that ddCTP encapsulated in erythrocytes is effective in inhibiting viral infectivity and replication in human and murine macrophages infected in vitro (12, 13). In vivo, a 3 month-treatment with ddCTP-loaded erythrocytes of mice infected with LP-BM5, reduced the typical signs of the disease (13). Other laboratories showed that

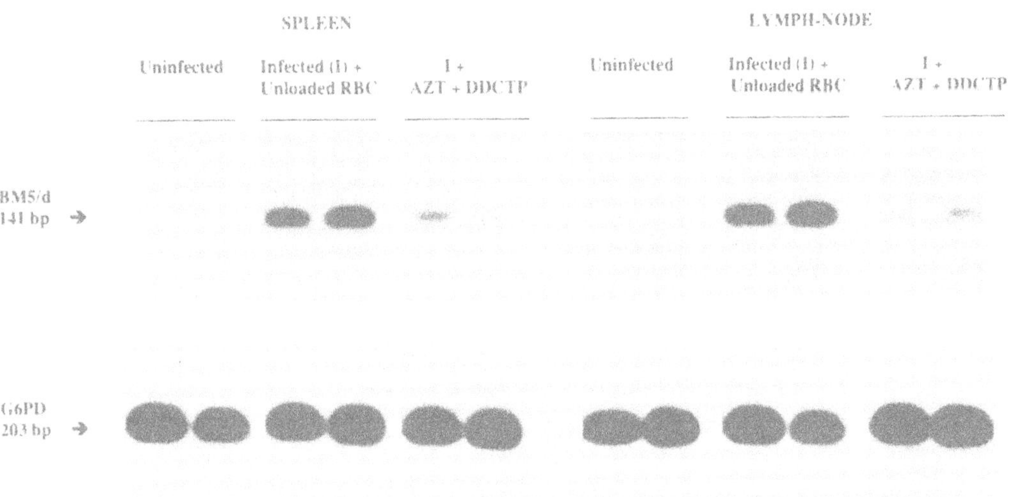

Figure 1. PCR detection of BM5d proviral DNA in the spleen and lymphonodes of C57BL/6 mice infected with LP-BM5 and treated with 250 mg/l of AZT in drinking water and ddCTP for 13 weeks. Results from two animals are shown. G6PD is an endogenous gene amplified as an internal control.

Table 3. Haematological parameters of LP-BM5 infected mice treated with AZT and erythrocytes ddCTP-loaded

	RBC (cells/μl)	Ht	MCV (fl)	MCH (pg/cell)	MCHC (g/dl)	HGB (g/dl)
Controls	8.125.000±387.675	36.7±1.8	42.0±0.9	17.7±0.4	39.2±1.2	14.4±0.4
Infected (I) + "unloaded" RBC	6.290.000±680.000	30.4±3.4	48.3±0.3	17.0±0.5	35.2±1.3	10.7±0.8
I+AZT+ddCTP	7.550.000±705.000	39.0±1.6	51.8±2.6	17.7±0.8	34.1±0.2	13.3±0.6

Values are means ± S.D. of 5 animals and have been obtained after 13 weeks of treatment

AZT treatment of C57BL/6 mice infected with LP-BM5 murine leukemia virus efficiently prevented the induction of immunodeficiency (14, 15). This regimen should protect both macrophages and lymphocytes. The results obtained show that the combination of erythrocytes ddCTP-loaded and AZT reduced some clinical signs of MAIDS but not all. In fact additive responses have been obtained in the reduction of splenomegaly, lymphoadenopathy and proviral DNA content. The hypergammaglobulinemia was reduced only after 7 weeks of treatment in animals receiving both treatments compared to those receiving the single treatment. No signs of toxicity have been observed in animals treated with AZT and erythrocytes ddCTP-loaded. The failure of nucleoside analogues, that inhibit viral reverse transcriptase, to reduce the circulating IgG in advanced stage of the disease can be due to the proliferation of B cells that undergo malignant transformation (4, 5). It will be interesting to use this animal model to experiment the combination of nucleoside analogues that can have a role on the number of cells that become infected with antineoplastic agents that act on the infected cells.

We can conclude that the antiretroviral regimen including drugs acting on different cell compartments is more effective than single drug in reducing some but not all the signs of MAIDS. Future experiments will evaluate the efficacy of combination of drugs acting at different levels of viral replication.

ACKNOWLEDGMENTS

This work was supported by Ministero della Sanità, Istituto Superiore della Sanità, Progetto AIDS 1996.

REFERENCES

1. Barrè-Sinoussi, F., J.C. Chermann, F. Rey, M.T. Nugeyre, S. Chamaret, J. Gruest, C. Dauget, C. Axler-Blin, F. Vezinet, C. Ronzioux, W. Rozembaum and L. Montagnier (1983). Isolation of a T-lymphotropic retrovirus from a patient at risk for acquired immunodeficiency syndrome (AIDS). Science, *220*, 868–871.
2. Popovic, M., M.G. Sarngadharan, E. Read and R.C. Gallo (1984). Detection, isolation, and continuous production of cytopathic retrovirus (HTLV-III) from patients with AIDS and pre-AIDS. Science, *224*, 497–501.
3. Mosier, D.E., R.A. Yetter and H.C. III Morse (1985). Retrovirus induction of acute lymphoproliferative disease and profound immunosuppression in adult C57BL/6 mice. J. Exp. Med. *61*, 767–772.
4. Morse, H.C. III, S.K. Chattopadhyay, N. Makino, T.N. Fredrickson, A.W. Hugin and J.W. Hartley (1992). Retrovirus-induced immunodeficiency in the mouse: MAIDS as a model for AIDS. AIDS *6*, 607–621.
5. Jolicoeur, P. (1991). Murine acquired immunodeficiency syndrome (MAIDS): an animal model to study the AIDS pathogenesis. Faseb J. *5*, 2398–2405.

6. Brandi, G., A. Casabianca, G.F. Schiavano, L. Rossi, A. Fraternale, A. Albano and M. Magnani (1995). Efficacy and toxicity of long-term administration of 2′,3′-dideoxycytidine in the LP-BM5 murine-induced immunodeficiency model. Antiv. Chem. & Chemother. *6(3)*, 153–161.
7. Rossi, L., G. Brandi, A. Fraternale, G.F. Schiavano, L. Chiarantini and M. Magnani (1993). Inhibition of murine retrovirus induced immunodeficiency disease by dideoxycytidine and dideoxycytidine 5′-triphosphate. J. of AIDS *6*, 1179–1186.
8. Yarchoan, R.K.M., J.A. Lietzau, B.-Y. Nygen, O.W. Brawley, J.M. Pluda, K.M. Wyvill, S.M. Steinberg, R. Agbaria, H. Mitsuya and S. Broder (1994). A randomized pilot study of alternating and simultaneous regimens of zidovudine (AZT) and didanosine (ddI) in patients with symptomatic human immunodeficiency virus (HIV) infection. J. Infect. Dis. *169*, 9–17.
9. Johnson, V.A., P. Merrill, T.C. Chou and M.S. Hirsch (1992). Human immunodeficiency virus type 1 (HIV-1) inhibitory interactions between protease inhibitor R. 31–8959 and zidovudine, 2′,3′-dideoxycytidine, or recombinant interferon alfa against zidovudine-sensitive or resistant HIV-1 in vitro. J. Infect. Dis. *166*, 1143–1146.
10. Gartner, S., P. Markovits, D.M. Markovits, M.H. Kaplan, R.C. Gallo and M. Popovic (1986). The role of mononuclear phagocytes in HTLV-III LAV infection. Science, *233*, 215–219.
11. Ho, D.D., T.R. Rota and M.S. Hirsch (1986). Infection of monocyte/macrophages by human T/lymphotropic virus type III. J. Clin. Invest., *77*, 12–15.
12. Magnani, M., A. Casabianca, L. Rossi, A. Fraternale, G. Brandi, L. Silvotti and G. Piedimonte (1995). Inhibition of HIV 1 and LP-BM5 replication in macrophages by dideoxycytidine and dideoxycytidine 5′-triphosphate. Antiv. Chem. & Chemother., *6(5)*, 312–319.
13. Magnani, M., L. Rossi, G. Brandi, G.F. Schiavano, M. Montroni and G. Piedimonte (1992). Targeting antiretroviral nucleoside analogues in phosphorylated form to macrophages: In vitro and in vivo studies. Proc. Natl. Acad. Sci., *89*, 6477–6481.
14. Ohnota, H., Y. Okada, H. Ushijima, T. Kitamura, K. Komuro and T. Mizuochi (1990). 3′-azido-3′-deoxythymidine prevents induction of murine acquired immunodeficiency syndrome in C57BL/10 mice infected with LP-BM5 murine leukemia viruses, a possible animal model for antiretroviral drug screening. Antimicr. Agents and Chemother., *34(4)*, 605–609.
15. Basham, T., C.D. Rios, T. Holdener and T.C. Merigan (1990). Zidovudine (AZT) reduces virus titer, retards immune dysfunction, and prolongs survival in the LP-BM5 murine induced immunodeficiency model. J. Infect. Dis. *161*, 1006–1009.
16. Mosier, D.E., R.A. Yetter and H.C. III Morse (1987). Functional T lymphocytes are required for a murine retrovirus induced immunodeficiency disease (MAIDS). J. Exp. Med., *165*, 1737–1742.
17. Aziz, D.C., Z. Hanna and P. Jolicoeur (1989). Severe immunodeficiency disease induced by a defective murine leukemia virus. Nature *338*, 505–508.
18. Kurdi-Haidar, B., P.J. Mason, A. Berrebi,G. Ankra-Badu, A. Al-Ali, A. Oppenheim and L. Luzzatto. (1990). Origin and spread of the glucose-6-phosphate dehydrogenase variant (G6PD-Mediterranean) in the Middle east. Am. J. Hum. Genet. *47*, 1013–1019.
19. Chattopadhyay, S.K., D.N. Sengupta, T.N. Fredrickson, H.C. III Morse and J.W. Hartley (1991). Characteristics and contributions of defective, ecotropic and mink cell focus-inducing viruses in a retrovirus induced immunodeficiency syndrome of mice. J. Virol., *65*, 4232–4241.

11

RED BLOOD CELLS AS A GLUCOCORTICOIDS DELIVERY SYSTEM

M. D'Ascenzo, A. Antonelli, L. Chiarantini, U. Mancini, and M. Magnani

Institute of Biological Chemistry "Giorgio Fornaini"
University of Urbino
Italy

1. INTRODUCTION

Macrophages are long-lived phagocytes with both cytocidal and microbicidal activity. These cells exist in a relatively quiescent basal state and also in "stimulated" or "activated" states. Activation of macrophages occurs by different stimuli (cytokines, bacterial lipopolysaccharide, etc.) and results in increased production of reactive oxygen metabolites and nitric oxide, increased phagocytic uptake, and release of many cytokines including IL-1, IL-6, TNF-α and growth factors (M-CSF, G-CSF). Upon activation macrophages also release lipid mediators (prostaglandins and leukotrienes) and numerous enzymes (1).

Inflammatory disorders are associated with the proliferation and activation of macrophages. In several cases the disease is induced by infections or drugs. In some cases (Langerhans cell histiocytosis) the etiology is unknown (2).

Glucocorticoid hormones are potent anti-inflammatory and immunosuppressive drugs (3).

Their action is mediated by suppression of cytokines production and TNF-α (3–9). In addition, glucocorticoids inhibit a number of macrophage functions associated with superoxide production and well known as "respiratory burst" (10). Based on these considerations we have evaluated the potential use of carrier erythrocytes as a drug-delivery and drug targeting systems for glucocorticoids analogues.

2. MATERIALS AND METHODS

2.1. Materials

Dexamethasone 21-phosphate (Dex-21-P), dexamethasone, prednisolone were from Sigma Chem.Co., prednisolone 21-phosphate (Pred-21-P) was a gift from Sochimia (Milan, Italy).

Erythrocytes as Drug Carriers in Medicine, edited by Sprandel and Way
Plenum Press, New York, 1997

2.2. Encapsulation of Dexamethasone-21-Phosphate and Prednisolone-21-Phosphate in Human Erythrocytes

Human blood was collected into heparinized tubes. Red blood cells (RBC) were isolated by centrifugation at 1,400 g at 4°C for 10 min from freshly drawn blood. The serum and buffy coat were removed and the packed cells were washed three times with 10 mM Hepes containing 140 mM NaCl, 5mM glucose, pH 7.4, and resuspended in the same buffer at a 70% hematocrit. Encapsulation of Dex-21-P or Pred-21-P in human erythrocytes was obtained by a procedure of hypotonic dialysis, isotonic resealing and reannealing essentially as reported in Ref. 11. Targeting of Dex-21-P-loaded erythrocytes to human macrophages was obtained by incubation of the drug-loaded cells with 1 mM $ZnCl_2$ and 1 mM bis(sulfosuccinimidyl)suberate

(BS^3) for 15 min at room temperature at an hematocrit of 10%. Further details are reported elsewhere (11).

2.3. Recognition of Drug-Loaded Erythrocytes by Macrophages

Mononuclear cells were prepared by Ficoll-Paque sedimentation from leukapheresed healthy donors, washed twice in sterile saline, and cultured in RPMI medium supplemented with 20% (vol/vol) heat inactivated human serum. After 24 h in culture, non adherent cells were removed and monocyte-derived macrophages were maintained in RPMI medium supplemented with 10% (vol/vol) fetal calf serum. Adherent cells (at least seven days of adherence) were incubated with Dex-21- P-loaded erythrocytes overnight at 37°C at a ratio of 100 erythrocytes per macrophage.

2.4. Cytofluorimetric Analysis

Aliquots of erythrocytes (5×10^5 cells) were resuspended in 25 µl of FITC-labelled anti-human IgG (Fc fragment) diluted 1:100 in 0.154 M NaCl, 5 mM NaH_2PO_4, pH 7.4, (PBS) or in FITC-labelled anti-C3 1:50 in PBS, both from Sigma Chem. Co.

After 30 min incubation at 4°C the cells were washed twice in PBS and resuspended to a final concentration of 1×10^5 ml^{-1} and used for cytofluorimetric analysis with a FACScan (Becton-Dickinson, Mountain View, CA).

2.5. Assay of Superoxide Anion Generation

Macrophages plated on a 35-mm-diameter plate were at a density of 2.5×10^5. Plated cells were quickly washed twice with PBS by vigorous swirling then the culture medium was replaced with the reaction mixture and the reaction was begun by placing the dishes in an incubator at 37°C in 5% CO_2 (95% air). The reaction mixture (final volume of 1 ml per dish) contained 80 µM cytocrome C, 20 mM Hepes and 5 mM glucose in PBS. O_2^- production was initiated by adding PMA 0.5 µM and opsonized latex beads. On addition of PMA the reaction mixture should be mixed and immediately added to plated cells to avoid inactivation of the PMA before contact is made with the macrophages. After 30 min incubation at 37°C the supernatants were used for spectrophotometric determinations. The OD550 nm of the reaction mixture is converted to nanomoles of cytochrome C reduced using the extinction coefficient $E_{550}=21 \times 10^3$ M^{-1} cm^{-1}.

2.6. Assay of TNF-α and IL-1β Production

Macrophages plated as above were stimulated with 10 μg/ml lipopolysaccarides from E.coli 0111:B4. TNF-α and IL-1β production in culture medium was determined 24 h later by ELISA assay kits from Boehringer Biochemica.

2.7. HPLC Chromatographic Determination of Dexamethasone and Prednisolone

Glucocorticoids analogues were determined by HPLC on boiled samples. Briefly, 0.1 vol. samples (resealed erythrocyte suspensions) were diluted with 0.9 vol of double distilled water, boiled for 5 min and filtered through 0.22 μm filters. This procedure allowed the recovery of > 95% of added Dex, Dex-21-P, Pred and Pred-21-P. HPLC chromatography was performed using a 5 μm Supelcosil LC-18 column (25 cm x 4.6 mm i.d.) protected by a guard column. The mobile phase consisted of two eluents: buffer A containing 10 mM KH_2PO_4, pH 5.0, and buffer B that consists of buffer A plus 70% v/v acetonitrile. The elution conditions were: 5 min 100% buffer A, up to 100% buffer B in 10 min and hold for 8 min. The gradient was returned to 100% buffer A in 3 min and initial conditions restored in 5 min. The flow-rate was 1.0 ml/min and detection was at 239 nm. Analyses were performed at room temperature and quantitative measurements were obtained by injection of standard of know concentration. The molar absorption value of corticosteroids studied at 239 nm was 14,000. The retention times under the conditions used were 17.4 min for Dex, 15.2 min for Dex-21-P, 14.33 min for Pred, and 8.62 min for Pred-21-P.

3. RESULTS

3.1. Dexametasone-21-Phosphate and Prednisolone-21-Phosphate Encapsulation in Human Erythrocytes

Dex-21-phosphate and Pred-21-phosphate were selected as non-diffusible glucocorticoid analogues to be encapsulated into erythrocytes. By a procedure of hypotonic dialysis and isotonic resealing we were able to internalize up to 10 μmoles of Dex-21-P per ml RBC. The main properties of loaded cells are reported in Table I.

Several properties of drug-loaded cells were investigated (ATP content, lactate production, etc.) and found to be unmodified.

3.2. Dexametasone-21-Phosphate and Prednisolone-21-Phosphate Stability

The stability of Dex-21-P and Pred-21-P was investigated both in drug-loaded erythrocytes and in human erythrocyte hemolysates. Dex-21-P encapsulated into human erythrocytes is converted to dexamethasone with t1/2 of 60± 1.8 h at 37°C. When Dex-21-P-loaded erythrocytes are stored at 4°C t1/2 was 6 ± 0.2 days. These values were obtained with Dex-21-P concentration in the loaded cells of 3 ±0.2 mM. Pred-21-P under similar conditions seems to be dephoshorylated faster then Dex-21-P. Definitive results are not jet available. In both cases drug-loaded cells were maintained at an hematocrit of 0.5% in RPMI-1640 medium contain-

Table 1. Some properties of Dexamethasone-21-P or Prednisolone 21-P loaded erythrocytes

	Dex-21-P	Predinisolone-21-P
Percentage encapsulation	30 ± 2%	28 ± 3%
Cell recovery	> 85%	> 85%
Mean cell volume	82 ± 1.5 fl	82 ± 2 fl
Highest concentration obtained	10 mM	6 mM

Values are mean ± S.D. of at least five experiments.

ing 10% heat-inactivated autologous serum. Concomitant to the decrease of Dex-21-P a stochiometric increase of Dexamethasone was found. Analyses of Dexamethsone in culture medium and in the intact cells provided similar values suggesting that the drug is in equilibrium between the intra and extra cellular compartments. The stability of Dex-21-P and Pred-21-P were investigated also in human erythrocyte lysates. Briefly, the erythrocyte hemolysate was first dialyzed overnight against 100 volumes of 0.9% (w/v) NaCl containing 10 mM $MgCl_2$, 10 mM Tris HCl, 0.02 mM EDTA, pH 7.5. The stability of Dex-21-P and Pred-21-P were investigated at 37°C and at a lysate concentration equivalent to 100 ± 8 mg hemoglobin/ml of incubation. Under these conditions both Dex-21-P and Pred-21-P are converted to the corresponding dephosphorylated glucocorticoid with a Km of 12.3 ± 0.4 mM and Vmax of 8 ± 0.3 nmoles/h/mg hemoglobin for Pred-21-P and a km of 11.1 ± 0.6 mM and Vmax of 7.4 ±0.2 nmoles/h/mg hemoglobin for Dex-21-P.

3.3. Targeting Dex-21-P-Loaded Erythrocytes to Macrophages

Targeting of drug-loaded RBC to macrophages was obtained by promoting the clusterization of the erythrocyte transmembrane protein band 3 (11). This clusterization was induced by the addition of 1 mM $ZnCl_2$ and BS^3. Zn is the clustering agent while BS^3 is a cross-linker that makes the clusters irreversible. Once formed these clusters are recognized by autologous immunoglobulins. In fact, treated erythrocytes once incubated for 15 min at 37°C in autologous serum are actively opsonized, and 92.7±1.1% become positive (by cytofluorimetric analyses) for surface bound IgG and 99.8±0.3% are also positive for C3b deposition. In other words the drug-loaded cells can now be recognized by macrophages though their Fc and C3b receptors. We have previously shown that erythrocytes treated as described above are actively phagocytosed (11). We have repeated these previous studies with Dex-21-P-loaded erythrocytes obtaining similar figures (1–1.2 RBC phagocytosed per macrophage after an overnight incubation; not shown). Thus, we have determined the amount of Dex-21-P transferred from Dex-21-P-loaded erythrocytes to macrophages. In three different experiments 5±0.9 nmol of Dex-21-P/10^6 macrophages were found after 12 h incubation of drug-loaded erythrocytes (3.5 μmol Dex-21-P/ml RBC) with macrophages at a ratio of 100 RBC/macrophage.

3.4. *In Vitro* Inhibition of Oxidative Burst

The respiratory burst can be elicited in macrophages with phorbol esters (which activate membrane-bound protein kinase C), and/or phagocytosis of opsonized latex particles. We have tested Dex-21-P-loaded erythrocytes as inhibitors of PMA and latex-activated oxidative burst. Since phagocytosis of drug-loaded RBC occurs during an overnight incubation of the erythrocytes with macrophages, and Dex-21-P encapsulated into RBC is not completely stable, we have performed preliminary experiments with Dex-21-P-loaded erythrocytes not treated with $ZnCl_2$ and BS^3. In other words, macrophages were incubated with Dex-21-P-loaded cells that were not modified to promote their opsonization and phagocytosis. By this way the dexamethasone eventually released into the culture medium during 12 h incubation (1.8 nmoles/ml culture medium) would eventually provide an inhibition comparable to that due to the release of dexamethasone by the Zn, BS^3 modified erythrocytes. In this control experiment, however, the inibition of oxidative burst was only 10–15% (range of three experiments) of O_2^- produced in the absence of drug-loaded erythrocytes. In contrast, Dex-21-P-loaded erythrocytes (3.5±0.2 μmol/ml RBC) produced a 60 to 70% inhibition of oxidative burst (Fig. 1).

3.5. Inhibition of TNF-α and IL-1β Production

Human macrophages when stimulated with bacterial lipopolysaccaride become activated and produce a number of cytokines. We have tested Dex-21-P- loaded erythrocytes for their ability to inhibit TNF-α and IL-1β production. As shown in Table II a potent supression of both TNF-α and IL-1β production was found.

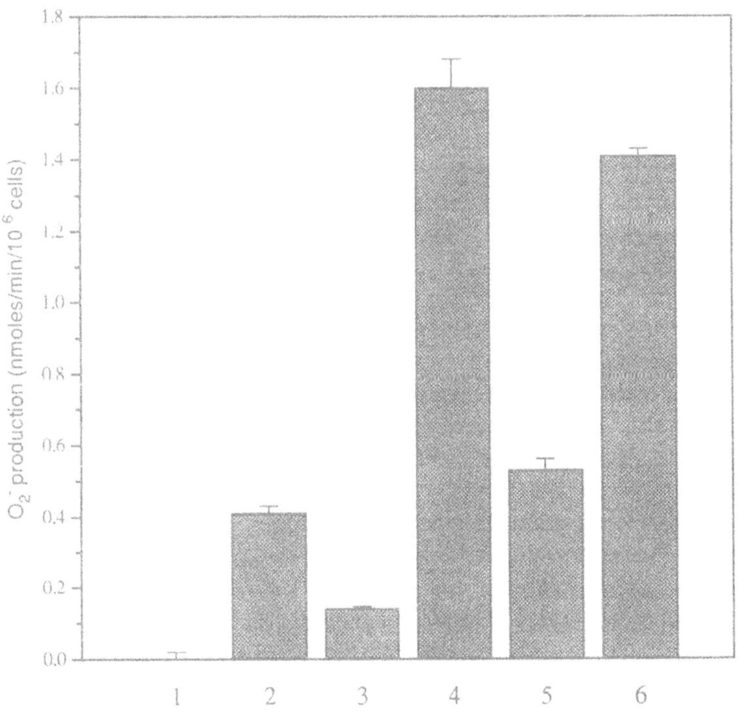

Figure 1. Inhibition of O_2^- production by Dexamethasone-21-phosphate loaded erythrocytes upon PMA stimulation. PMA was 0.5 μM for 30 min; Dex-21-P in macrophages was 5 ± 0.9 nmoles/10^6 cells; Dex in solution was 1.8 nmoles/ml corresponding to the calculated amount of drug eventually released by Dex-21-P loaded erythrocytes. 1, control macrophages; 2, PMA stimulated macrophages; 3, macrophages receiving Dex-21-P-loaded erythrocytes stimulated by PMA; 4, macrophages receiving PMA and latex beads; 5, macrophages receiving Dex-21-P-loaded erythroytes and stimulated with PMA and latex beads; 6, macrophages stimulated with PMA, latex beads and receiving dexamethasone in solution.

Table 2. Inhibition of human macrophages TNF-α and IL-1 β production by free and encapsulated Dexamethasone-21-phosphate

Cells	TNF-α production * ng/10^5 cells/24 h	IL-1 β production ** pg/10^5 cells/24 h
Macrophages	ND	ND
Macrophages + LPS (10 μg/ml) [a]	80 ± 10	169
Macrophages + LPS + UL-RBC [b]	85 ± 9	134
Macrophages + LPS + L-RBC [c]	25 ± 9	28
Macrophages + LPS + Dex 1 μM in medium	31 ± 10	ND
Macrophages + LPS + Dex 0.1 μM in medium	28 ± 8	ND

ND, not detectable.
[a]LPS, endotoxic lipopolysaccarides from Escherichia coli 0111: B4
[b]UL-RBC, unloaded erythrocytes
[c]L-RBC, loaded erythrocytes (0.3 μmoles Dexamethasone- 21-P/ml erythrocytes)
*values are the mean ± S.D. of four experiments
**values are the mean of two experiments that agreed within 12%

4. DISCUSSION

Glucocorticoid hormones because of their inhibition of cytokines release and other macrophage functions are widely used anti-inflammatory and immunosupressive drugs (3). The results reported in this paper show that both Dexamethasone-21-phosphate and Prednisolone-21-phosphate can be easily entrapped into human erythrocytes where they are slowly dephosphorylated to the corresponding glucocorticoid by erythrocyte resident enzymes. This slow de-phosphorylation rate suggest at least two possible uses of glucocorticoid loaded erythrocytes. The carrier cells can perform as slow delivery systems fo the release of the corticosteroids or, when properly modified by band 3 clustering, they can perform as a drug targeting systems for the selective delivery of Dex-21-P or Pred-21-P into macrophages. In Fig. 2 we have simulated the *in vivo* pharmacokinetic of blood dexamethasone when injected intravenously or administered as dexamethasone-21-P in autologous erythrocytes. It is worth noting that to maintain a drug concentration within therapeutic values the drug should be repeatidly administered at 3.5 hours intervals while a single administration of drug loaded cells will provide similar blood concentrations of the drug for several days. It can be also easily calculated that the total drug concentration administered by carrier erythrocytes is less then half the total amount of drug administered free to obtain similar "area under the curve".

The second interesting application of glucocorticoid-loaded erythrocytes concern the possibility of using these cells for the selective delivery of glucocorticoids to macrophages. Macrophages are involved in a number of diseases including inflammatory disorders. Due to the high rate of sequestration of carrier erythrocytes modified by the membrane remodelling procedure described above (11) it seems reasonable to suggest their use for local (i.e. intra-articular) administration. Liposomes entrapped drugs (12, 13) have already shown an increased retention of the drug in the injected joint.

In conclusion, the red blood cell seems to be extremely useful carriers for both a slow release of glucocorticoids or the targeted administration of these drugs to resident macrophages where high concentrations could be attained with minimal systemic toxicity. The "*in vivo*" preliminary data already obtained in our laboratory support the above conclusions.

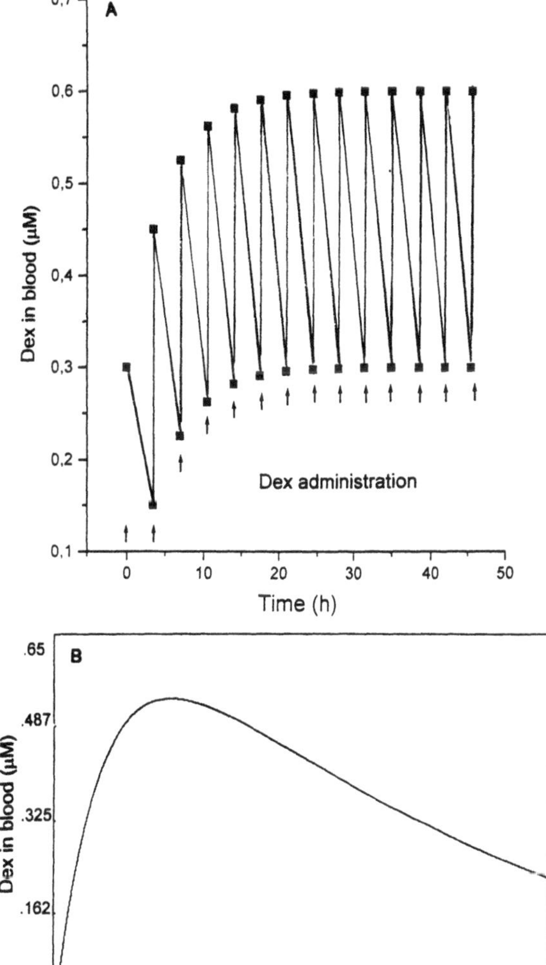

Figure 2. Simulated *in vivo* pharmacokinetic of dexamethasone when administered (A) at 3.5 hours intervals at a 0.01 mg/Kg body weight in a 70 Kg human being or (B) when administered encapsulated into 10 ml of autologous erythrocytes containing 3 μmoles of dexamethasone-21-phosphate per ml erythrocytes. The *in vivo* t1/2 for glucocorticoids is ≅ 3 hours.

ACKNOWLEDGMENTS

This work was partially supported by M.U.R.S.T. and C.N.R. founds.

REFERENCES

1. Horton, M.A. (ed.) (1993). Blood Cell Biochemistry. 5. Macrophages and related cells. Plenum Press, New York, pp. 434.
2. Lichtman, M.A., Komp, D.M. (1995). Inflammatory and malignant histiocytosis. In: Williams Hematology (E. Beutler, M.A. Lichtman, B.S. Coller and T.J. Kipps eds) Mc Graw-Hill, Inc., New York, pp. 885.
3. Haynes,R.C. (1990) Adrenocorticotropic hormons: Adrenocortical steroids and their synthetic analogs: Inhibition of the synthesis and actions of adrenocortical hormones, in "Goodman and Gilman's: The Pharmacological Basis of Therapeutics" (Gilman, A.G., rall, T.W., Nies, A.S., Tylor, P. Eds) pp 1431–1457, Pergamon, New York:

4. Snyder, D.S., Unanue, U.R. (1982). Corticosteroids inhibit murine macrophage Ia expression and interleukin I production. J. Immunol. 129, 1803–1805.
5. Lew, W., Oppenheim, J.J., Matsushima, K. (1988). Analysis of the suppression of IL-1α and 1β production in human peripheral blood mononuclear adherent cells by a glucocorticoid hormone. J. Immunol. 140, 1895–1901.
6. Tobler, A., Meier, R., Seitz, M., Dewald, B., Baggiolini, M., Fey, M.F. (1992). Glucocorticoids downregulate gene expression of GM-CSF, NAP-1/IL-8, and IL-6 but not of M-CSF in human fibroblasts. Blood 79, 45–51.
7. Culpepper, J.A., Lee, F. (1985). Regulation of IL3 expression by glucocorticoids in cloned murine T lymphocytes. J. Immunol. 135, 3191–3197.
8. Gadina, M., Bertini,R., Mengozzi, M., Zandalasini, M., Montovani, A., Ghezzi, P. (1992). Protective effect of chlorpromazine on endotoxin toxicity and TNF production in glucocorticoid sensitive and glucocorticoid-resistant models of endotoxic shock. J. Exp. Med. 173,1305–1310.
9. Beutler, B., Krochin, N., Milsark, I.W., Luedke, C., Cerami A. (1986). Control of cachectin (tumor necrosis factor) synthesis: Mechanisms of endotoxin resistance. Science 232, 977–979.
10. Maridonneau-Parini, I., Errasfa, M. and Russo-Marie, F. (1989). Inhibition of O_2^- generation by dexamethasone is mimicked by lipocortin I in alveolar macrophages. J. Clin. Invest. 83, 1936–1940.
11. Magnani, M., Rossi, L., Brandi, G., Schiavano, G.F., Montroni, M. and Piedimonte G. (1992). Targeting antiretroviral nucleoside analogues in phosphorylated form to macrophages: *in vitro* and *in vivo* studies. Proc. Natl. Acad. Sci. U.S.A. 83, 6477–6481.
12. Dingle, J.T. (1976). Liposomes in the treatment of inflammatory joint disease. In: Gordon, I.L., Hazelman, B.L. (eds) Reumatoid Arthrities: Cellular pathology and pharmacology. Elsevier, Amsterdam, pp. 259–266.
13. Foong, W.C. and Green, K.L. (1983). treatment of antigen-induced arthritis in rabbits with liposome-entrapped methotrexate injected intra-articularly. J. Pharm. Pharmacol. 45, 204–209.

12

ORGANOPHOSPHORUS ANTAGONISM BY RESEALED ERYTHROCYTES CONTAINING RECOMBINANT PARAOXONASE

J. L. Way, L. Pei, I. Petrikovics, D. McGuinn, C. Tamulinas, Q. Z. Hu, E. P. Cannon, and A. Zitzer

Department of Medical Pharmacology and Toxicology
Texas A&M University Health Science Center
College Station, Texas, 77843–1114

ABSTRACT

Parathion has the highest incidence of poisonings among the agricultural pesticides. An alternative conceptual approach was employed to prevent intoxication of paraoxon, the active metabolite of parathion, by using resealed carrier erythrocytes containing a highly purified recombinant paraoxonase (CRBC). The CRBC were found to be effective alone and synergistic with 2-PAM and atropine to protect over 1,000 lethal doses of paraoxon. This striking protection greatly exceeds any antidotal regimen ever reported against chemical toxicants. The present drug carrier model provides a general conceptual approach to develop specific antidotes against many other chemical toxicants for which no antidotes are presently available.

INTRODUCTION

Organophosphorus (OP) insecticides are the most widely used agricultural pesticides and parathion is the most prevalent organophosphorus agent currently employed. As would be expected, more morbidity and mortality have been attributed to parathion than any other agricultural pesticides[1]. Its toxicity is due to the biotransformation to the more toxic metabolite, paraoxon. The mechanism of OP intoxication is due to the inhibition of acetylcholinesterase (AChE), thereby causing an excessive accumulation of acetylcholine[2]. Specific antidotes for OP poisoning are atropine and pralidoxime (2-PAM). Atropine competitively blocks the pharmacological effect of acetylcholine at he muscarinic receptor[3] and 2-PAM reactivates OP-inhibited acetylcholinesterase[4]. However, neither of these two antidotes actually degrades the OP agent. The present approach is to directly hydrolyze the toxicant using highly purified recombinant paraoxonase[5] encapsulated within

Erythrocytes as Drug Carriers in Medicine, edited by Sprandel and Way
Plenum Press, New York, 1997

annealed resealed carrier erythrocytes (CRBC) prepared by hypotonic dialysis. These CRBCs are far superior in protecting against the lethal effects of paraoxon than the classic antidotal combination of 2-PAM and atropine[4]. Moreover, when 2-PAM and atropine was administered in combination with CRBC, a striking synergism occurred, as the protection was over 1000 lethal doses (LD_{50}) of paraoxon. This protective effect greatly exceeds our expectation, as there are less then five specific antidotes which can protect over three LD_{50} doses of any chemical toxicants.

MATERIALS AND METHODS

Male Balb/cAnNcrlBR mice weighing between 18–25 g were distributed randomly into experimental groups and the effects of various treatments on the lethality of paraoxon were assessed. All animal procedures were conducted in accordance with the NIH Guide for the Care and Use of Laboratory Animals. The LD_{50} values which were based on 24-hour mortality, were determined in five or more groups that contained eight or more mice each. The LD_{50} values of these experiments were analyzed according to the method of Litchfield and Wilcoxon[6] as adapted to the computer program PHARM/PCS version 4.2 [7].

Paraoxonase purified from *E. Coli* expression cells carrying *opd* gene cloned from *Flavobacterium spp.* was encapsulated within murine carrier erythrocytes. The resealed annealed carrier erythrocytes were prepared as following: Blood samples from Balb/C mice were collected and white blood cells were removed by centrifugation. Erythrocytes were collected and mixed with purified enzyme. The mixture was placed under a hypotonic condition (50 mOsm/kg) to dialyze for 30–40 minutes. Dialysis was continued until osmolarity reached 130–150 mOsm/kg. After equilibration for 30 minutes, the erythrocytes were resealed by adding 9% NaCl and annealed at 37°C. After washing several times with phosphate buffer, these carrier cells are ready for intravenous administration.

RESULTS

Doses and routes of administration of the antagonists are given in Table 1. Carrier erythrocytes, atropine and 2-PAM were administered 60, 30 and 15 minutes, respectively, prior to the administration of paraoxon. The protective effect of the carrier erythrocytes, atropine and 2-PAM, either alone or in combination in antagonizing paraoxon intoxication are expressed as LD_{50} values (Table 1). The administration of paraoxon in vehicle control animals gave an LD_{50} value of 0.95 mg/kg. A protection was observed in animals treated with atropine and 2-PAM as the LD_{50} value of paraoxon was elevated to 53.7 mg/kg (Experiment 2). Employment of CRBCs was nor only effective in antagonizing paraoxon intoxication as indicated by an LD_{50} value of 119.9 mg/kg of paraoxon (Experiment 3) but also considerably more efficacious than the classic antidotal treatment of atropine and 2-PAM. Furthermore, mice receiving CRBCs did not show any signs of OP intoxication at dose levels that were lethal to the classic antidotal combination of atropine and 2-PAM. A striking synergistic effect was observed when these antagonists were administered in combination, as the LD_{50} value was elevated to 991.2 mg/kg (Experiment 4) which was over 1,000 times the LD_{50} value of paraoxon.

Potency ratios are often used in pharmacology/toxicology to compare the efficacy of various treatments (Table 1). It is a term derived by dividing LD_{50} value of paraoxon with antagonist(s) by the LD_{50} value of paraoxon without antagonist(s). Respective slopes of

Table 1. Effect of Atropine, 2-PAM, and CRBC paraoxonase on the LD50 of paraoxon in mice[a]

Exp.	Treatment before paraoxon	Slope Function	LD_{50} (mg/kg)[b] (limits, p=0.5)	Potency Ratios
1	Control	1.34	0.95 (0.84 - 1.08)	1.0
2	ATR[c] + 2-PAM	1.24	53.67 (44.89-64.16)*	56.5
3	CRBC	1.47	119.9 (91.2 - 157.6)*	126.2
4	CRBC+ATR+PAM	1.20	991.2 (891.4 - 1103.2)*	1042.4

[a]Paraoxon (0.6 to 1,200 mg/kg) was delivered subcutaneously to mice in 6% cyclodextrin and/or propylene glycjol solvent solutions. The Propylene glycol solvent consisted of 40% propylene glycol, 10% ethanol, and 50% water. Atropine sulfate (10 mg/kg) and 2-PAM-Cl (90 mg/kg) was given intraperitoneally. CRBC (0.2 ml/mice was given intraveneously through tail vein.
[b]Each LD50 value was obtained from 5 or more graded doses of paraoxon administered to 5 or more groups of 8 or more mice/group.
[c]ATR = atropine sulfate.
*Significantly different from control.

the dose-response mortality curve for each experiment employing paraoxon and/or its antagonists were found not to be significantly different from that of paraoxon alone; thus, comparisons of the potency ratios are valid. The potency ratio of the control group (without antagonists) is regarded as one. Atropine sulfate and 2-PAM raised the potency ratio to 56.5. CRBC alone is more effective than the classic antidotes as the potency ratio was 126.2. A striking protective effect was also observed when CRBC were used in combination with atropine sulfate and 2-PAM as the potency ratio was increased to 1042.4.

DISCUSSION

Attempts to degrade OPs by administering the free enzyme directly into the bloodstream have been reported[8]. However, the use of free enzyme presents major problems due to the massive amount of enzyme required and the short duration of action. These shortcomings can be circumvented by placing the enzymes in a protected bioenvironment such as resealed erythrocytes, which would prolong the duration of action of these enzymes[9]. This prompted studies on encapsulation of various OP hydrolyzing enzymes within carrier cells[10]. Carrier erythrocytes containing recombinant paraoxonase were employed as a model to represent a new approach in preventing OP intoxication. Moreover, the use of CRBC with the classic antidotal combination provided the highest antidotal efficacy ever reported against any chemical toxicants. This increased protective effect can be attributed to various factors: Firstly, CRBC would lower blood paraoxon concentration, as the CRBC would degrade the toxicant as soon as it enters the bloodstream, resulting in less severe AChE inhibition. Secondly, CRBC would increase the efficacy of atropine, as atropine competitively blocks acetylcholine at eh muscarinic receptor sites. Finally, CRBC would increase 2-PAM efficacy in reactivating paraoxon-inhibited AChE, as aging of the AChE is minimized. Aging of OP-inhibited AChE usually presents a major obstacle to reactivation of the enzyme during treatment of OP poisoning, as once aging occurs, 2-PAM and other reactivators are no longer effective.

These carrier cells may be useful in preventing organophosphorus induced delayed and chronic neurotoxicity (OPIDN)[4]. Development of OPIDN may be partially attributed to the redistribution of OP from fat depot as most OPs tend to distribute and store in adipose tissues.

When exposure is terminated, the fat tissue may serve as a reservoir to continuously release OPs into the blood. By placing paraoxonase within the circulation, this enzyme can constantly remove OP which is being slowly released into the blood stream from fatty tissues, thereby minimizing the incidence of OPIDN.

This general approach serves as a model to provide the impetus to develop effective specific antidotes, which are now almost nonexistent, against numerous chemical intoxicants by the application of a combination of molecular biology and carrier system biotechnology.

REFERENCES

1. W. J. Hayes, W. K. Vaughn, *Toxicol. Appl. Pharmacol.* **42**, 235 (1977).
2. G. Schrader, *Angew. Chem.* **61**, 471 (1950).
3. W. Modell, S. Krop, *J. Pharmacol. Exp. Ther.* **88**, 34 (1946).
4. I.B. Wilson, S. Ginsburg, *Arch. Biochem. Biophys.* **54**, 569 (1955).
5. C. S. Steven, L. L. Harper, J. R. Wild, *J. Bacteriol.* **170**, 2306 (1988). Synonyms: paraoxonase, organophosphorus acid anhydrase, parathion hydrolase, parathion arylesterase, and arylalkylphosphatase (EC 3.1.8.1) . E. Beiner, *Chem. -Biol. Intereactions.* **87**, 15 (1993). G.A. Omburo, J. M. Kuo, L.S. Mullins, F. M. Raushel. *J. Biol. Chem.* **267**, 13278 (1992). W. W. Mulbry, J. S. Karns, *J. Bacteriol.* **171**, 6740 (1989).
6. J. T. Litchfield, Jr., F. Wilcoxon, *J. Pharmacol. Exp. Ther.* **96**, 99 (1949).
7. R.J. Tallarida, R.B. Murray, *Manual of Pharmacologic Calculations with Computer Program.* (Springer-Verlag, New York ed. 2, 1987).
8. J. M. Cohen,, M. G. P. J. Warringa, *Biochim. Biophys. Acta.* **26**, 29 (1957); Y. Ashani, N. Rothshild, Y. Segall, D. Levanon, L. Raveh, *Life Sci.* **49**, 367 (1991); C. A. Broomfield. *Chem.-Biol. Interactions.* **87**, 297 (1993).
9. G. M. Ihler, R. H. Glew, F. W. Schnure, *Proc. Natl. Acad. Sci. USA*, **70**, 2663 (1973); DeLoach, J. R.. *Medicinal Research Review* **6**, 487 (1986); P. Leung, W. D. Davis, C. C. Yao, E. P. Cannon, J. L. Way. *Fundam. Appl. Toxicol.* **16**, 559–661 (1991).
10. W. D. McGuinn et al., *Fundam. Appl. Toxicol.* **21**, 38 (1993); L. Pei et al., *Fundam. Appl. Toxicol.* **124**, 296 (1994). L. Pei et al., *Biochem. Appl. Biotech.*, in press.
11. M. Lotti, *Critical Rev. in Toxicol.* **21**, 465 (1992).
12. This study was supported by funds from Texas A&M University, USARMDC and NIEHS. We are grateful to Jennifer McNamee for her assistance in the preparation of this manuscript.

13

BIOTINYLATION OF ERYTHROCYTES PREPARES TO ALLOW CIRCULATION-STABLE IMMUNOERYTHROCYTES CAPABLE OF RECOGNIZING THE ANTIGEN

Juan C. Murciano,[1] Vladimir R. Muzykantov,[2] and Angel Herráez[1]

[1]Department of Biochemistry and Molecular Biology
University of Alcalá de Henares
Spain
[2]Institute for Environmental Medicine
University of Pennsylvania
Philadelphia, Pennsylvania

1. INTRODUCTION

Erythrocytes (RBC) have been studied as carriers of drugs for several years[3]. Their viability, physiologic characteristics and the availability of different procedures to incorporate substances into them support their utilization[10]. However, targeting is one of the major problems to solve in all these related therapies. Attachment of antibodies to the RBC surface has been pursued before[2]. This attachment may provide a way to target these carriers to the specific zone where the disease is, and also can serve as a means to eliminate hazardous antigens from the bloodstream. Biotin/streptavidin (b/SAv) complex is one of the systems to attach antibodies or other substances, such as enzymes, to the RBC surface[5,9]. Although there are several works which have proposed the development of immunoerythrocytes, little is known about their ability to recognize the antigen after their circulation in the animal model. Looking for these topics, in this work we investigate the attachment of biotinylated antibody (b-Ab) to biotinylated RBC by means of bridging SAv molecules. We show that moderate biotinylation of the RBC allows to attach 3 to 5 $x10^4$ molecules of b-Ab and creates immunoerythrocytes that are stable in circulation. The b-Ab remains attached to the RBC while they are circulating. Furthermore, the immunoerythrocytes entirely retain the ability to recognize the antigen.

Erythrocytes as Drug Carriers in Medicine, edited by Sprandel and Way
Plenum Press, New York, 1997

2. MATERIALS AND METHODS

6-biotinylaminocaproic acid N-hydroxysuccinimide ester (long arm biotin ester, BxNHS), streptavidin and polyclonal goat antibody against mouse IgG were purchased from Calbiochem. Normal mouse IgG, bovine serum albumin (BSA) and dimethylformamide (DMF) were from Sigma. $Na^{51}CrO_4$ and $Na^{125}I$ isotopes were bought from Amersham. Proteins were radiolabelled with ^{125}I by the Iodogen method (Pierce) according to the manufacturer's recommendations. Goat antibody against mouse IgG was biotinylated with BxNHS by standard method[1].

Sprague-Dawley male rats weighing 250–300 g were anesthetized with i.p. injection of sodium pentobarbital (50 mg/Kg). To obtain RBC, blood was collected from descending aorta in heparin. RBC pellet was washed 4 times with PBS. Biotinylation was performed by incubation of 10% suspensions of RBC in borate buffer, pH 9.0, with BxNHS in DMF at different micromolar concentrations (which are expressed as b_n in the text). After 30 min at room temperature, the RBC were washed four times by centrifugation with BSA-PBS (1 mg/ml BSA in PBS). Streptavidin (SAv) was added to 10% suspension of b-RBC ($1x10^6$ SAv molecules per RBC) and after 30 minutes incubation at room temperature non-bound SAv was removed by 3 washes. In a separate experiment, radioiodinated SAv was used in order to estimate SAv binding.

Immunoerythrocytes were prepared as previously described[6]: Biotinylated anti-IgG (b-Ab) was attached to b_{20}RBC/SAv by incubation of b-Ab ($2x10^5$ molecules per RBC) with 10% suspension of b-RBC/SAv for 1 hour at room temperature. Non-bound b-Ab was eliminated by 3 washes with BSA-PBS. Radiolabelled b-Ab was used as a tracer in a separate experiment to estimate the b-Ab attachment to the b-RBC/SAv.

To trace immunoerythrocytes after *in vivo* administration, ^{51}Cr isotope was added to b_{20}RBC/SAv suspension simultaneously with either b-Ab or ^{125}I-b-Ab and incubated for 1 hour at room temperature. Excess of Cr was eliminated by centrifugation. Efficiency of RBC radiolabelling was 35–50%. Experiments in animals were designed as described earlier[8]. Briefly, $5x10^7$ ^{51}Cr-immunoerythrocytes were injected through the tail vein to anesthetized rats. At indicated times after injection, rats were sacrificed by exsanguination. Blood and internal organs were collected, and the latter were rinsed in saline to eliminate blood. ^{51}Cr and ^{125}I in blood (pellet fraction after centrifugation at 500 g) and organs were measured in a gamma-counter.

To study the antigen recognition by the immunoerythrocytes, $5x10^7$ ^{51}Cr-labelled b_{20}RBC/SAv/b-Ab were similarly injected, and after 1 hour animals were sacrificed by exsanguination. 1 ml of blood was then incubated with ^{125}I-labelled mouse IgG. As a control, the immunoerythrocytes that had not been injected were diluted with normal blood and 1 ml was incubated as well with the radiolabelled mouse IgG. After 1 hour, non-bound IgG was washed off by centrifugation 4 times with BSA-PBS. ^{51}Cr and ^{125}I associated to RBC were measured in a gamma-counter.

3. RESULTS

Figure 1 shows the progressive attachment of SAv to RBC treated with increasing concentrations of biotin. The total amount of SAv added was kept constant at $1x10^6$ molecules. It can be seen that attachment of b-Ab to these b-RBC/SAv correlates with that of SAv binding, except for the highest concentration of biotin (b_{700}RBC) for which the ability to bind b-Ab decreases.

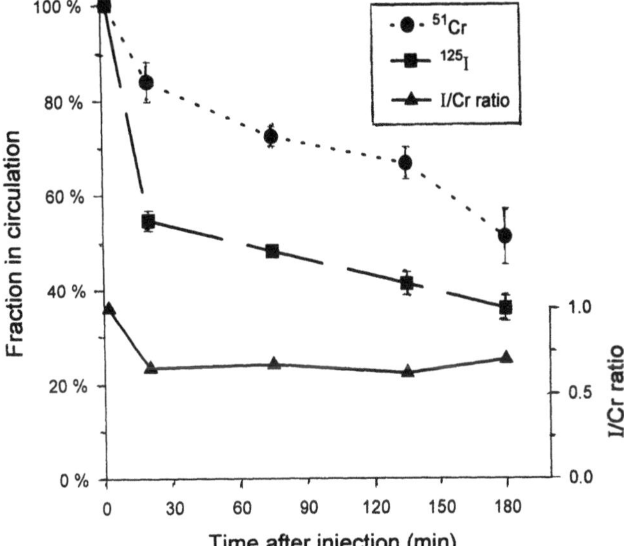

Figure 1. Binding of streptavidin and subsequent binding of biotinylated antibody to RBC biotinylated with increasing concentrations of BxNHS. Filled circles and left axis: ^{125}I-SAv bound to b_nRBC. Hollow squares and right axis: ^{125}I-b-Ab bound to b_nRBC/SAv.

Figure 2 demonstrates circulation of immunoerythrocytes in the animal model. Both radiolabels, ^{51}Cr for the RBC and ^{125}I for the attached b-Ab, follow similar profiles. The ratio between both isotopes shows that there is only a decrease of iodine with respect to chromium in the first 15 minutes, and no subsequent loss of iodine from the RBC. The value of this ratio is close to 70% of that in the injected preparation, which indicates the maintenance of the biotinylated antibody in circulation attached to the mildly biotinylated RBC. Lastly, the ^{51}Cr pattern indicates an acceptable circulation (60%) of the modified RBC population at least up to 3 hours after injection.

Figure 3 studies the biodistribution of Cr and I isotopes at 1 hour and 3 hours after injection of b_{20}RBC/SAv/b-Ab immunoerythrocytes in the rats. As a control, it is also

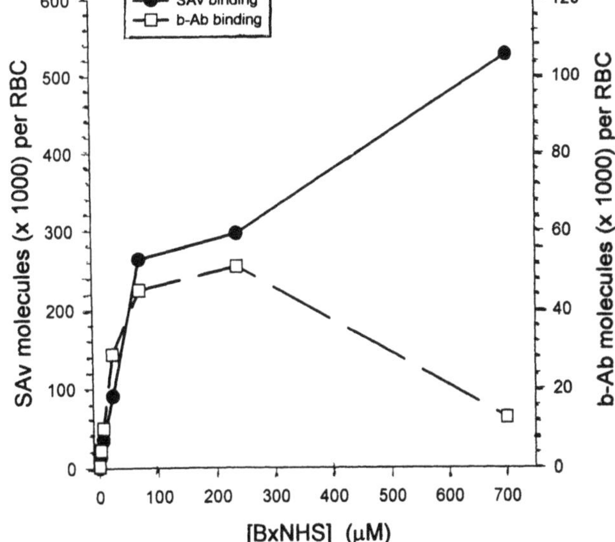

Figure 2. *In vivo* kinetics of ^{51}Cr-RBC and ^{125}I-antibody in b_{20}RBC/SAv/b-Ab immunoerythrocytes. Circles and left axis: ^{51}Cr associated to RBC (% of injected dose). Squares and left axis: ^{125}I-b-Ab attached to RBC (% of injected dose). Triangles and right axis: ratio between ^{125}I and ^{51}Cr associated to RBC, expressed relative to injected sample. (Mean ± SD, n=3)

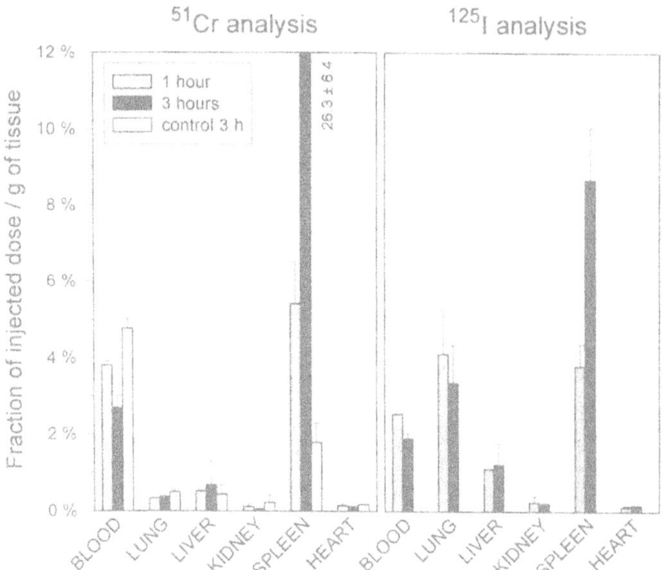

Figure 3. Biodistribution of ^{51}Cr-RBC (left panel) and ^{125}I-antibody (right panel) in b_{20}RBC/SAv/b-Ab immunoerythrocytes. Radioactivity in blood and organs 1 hour (hatched bars) and 3 hours (filled bars) after injection of immunoerythrocytes is made relative to injected dose and expressed per gram of tissue. Control was ^{51}Cr-labeled, non-biotinylated RBC after 3 hours (hollow bars). (Mean ± SD, n=3)

shown the biodistribution of naive (non-biotinylated) chromium-labeled cells at 3 hours. As already observed in the previous figure, about 50% of Cr radioactivity remains in circulation. The only organ with an increased uptake of immunoerythrocytes, as compared to control, is spleen and especially at 3 hours after injection. This indicates a partial elimination of these immunoerythrocytes. However, there is still a major proportion of them in blood. The iodine counts show a similar distribution in most of the organs studied except for its accumulation in the lung.

Figure 4 compares the I/Cr ratios in blood and organs at 1 hour and 3 hours and complements the data presented in previous figure. The ratios remain constant and in the range close to1 in most of the organs except for the lung, where an accumulation of b-Ab with respect to RBC is observed.

Figure 5 presents the capacity of the immunoerythrocytes, after their circulation for 1 hour *in vivo*, to bind the antigen (mouse IgG). This is compared to that of immunoerythrocytes that have not been injected. In separate experiments, using ^{125}I-b-Ab, the amount of antibody attached to RBC was measured. Inset in Fig. 5 shows that the antigen (IgG) bound is proportional to the actual amount of b-Ab attached to the b_{20}RBC/SAv.

4. DISCUSSION

The present study proposes long-circulating immunoerythrocytes that are able to recognize efficiently the antigen after circulation.

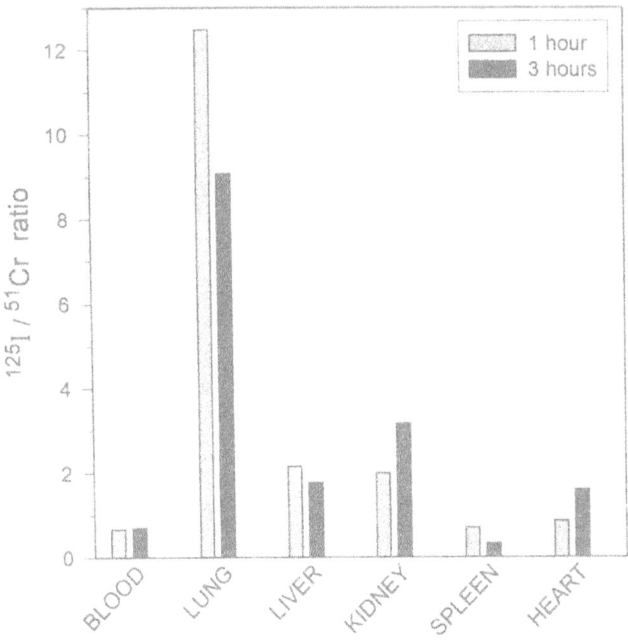

Figure 4. Ratio between ^{125}I-antibody and ^{51}Cr-RBC and labels in blood and organs after i.v. injection of ^{51}Cr-b_{20}RBC/SAv/^{125}I-b-Ab complex. Ratios presented are calculated from data in Fig. 3.

By changing the concentration of biotin ester, increasing amounts of SAv can be bound to the RBC surface (Fig. 1). Subsequent attachment of biotinylated antibody correlates with the level of SAv, except for the highest concentration of biotin tested (700 μM), where there is a drop in the amount of b-Ab bound. This is probably due to multivalent attachment of SAv molecules to the biotin residues on the RBC surface, reducing the number of sites available for b-Ab binding. Previous studies have shown that high concentrations of biotin ester lead, after SAv binding, to RBC lysis in the presence of serum, and this can also be explained by the multivalent binding of SAv molecules, with clustering of biotinylated surface proteins, including complement regulators[11].

Successful use of RBC modification by the biotin/SAv system requires an important characteristic: maintenance of the physiologic behavior of the cell. To this purpose, low concentrations of the biotin ester (20 μM) have been shown to produce circulation-stable b-RBC/SAv complexes[7]. In addition, these b_{20}RBC/SAv attach enough b-Ab molecules (approx. 30000) as it is shown in Fig. 1.

Kinetics and biodistribution of these immunoerythrocytes show their fate in the circulation up to 3 hours (Fig. 2 and Fig. 3, blood ^{51}Cr values). In addition, the b-Ab remains attached to the carrier cells, as is expressed by the constancy of the ratio between the ^{125}I-label of the b-Ab and the ^{51}Cr-label of the RBC (Fig. 2). Despite this fair persistence in circulation, there is a loss of approximately 30% of the b-Ab during the first minutes after the inoculation (Fig. 2), which likely corresponds to easily detachable proteins (such as GPI-anchored proteins[4,11]) that were biotinylated on the RBC surface. This detached b-Ab molecules accumulate in the lung, as it is reflected by their label (Fig. 3), probably be-

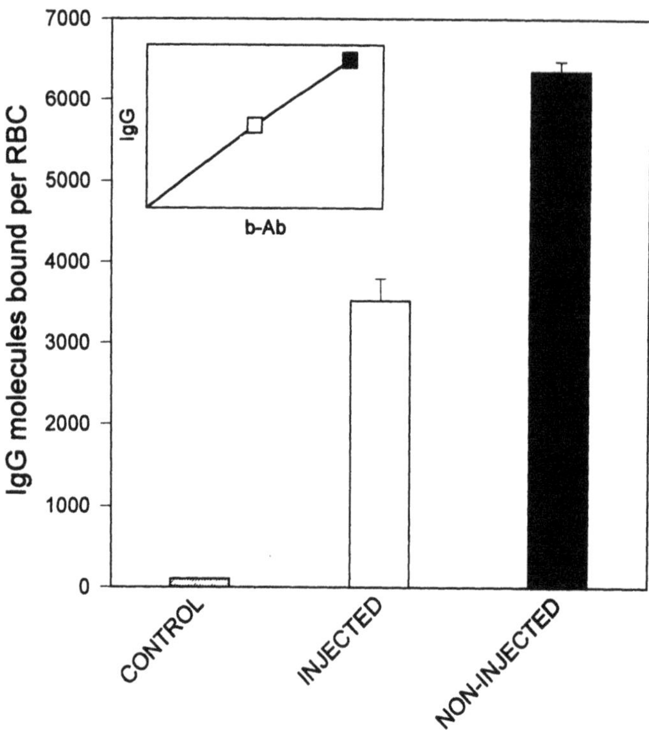

Figure 5. Recognition of antigen (mouse IgG) by immunoerythrocytes (b_{20}RBC/SAv/b-Ab). Inset graphic represents relation and between b-Ab and IgG in the immunoerythrocytes samples. Hatched bars: ^{51}Cr-RBC incubated with the antigen (^{125}I-IgG). Hollow bar and square: ^{51}Cr-b_{20}RBC/SAv/b-Ab extracted after 1 hour in circulation incubated with the antigen. Filled bar and square: ^{51}Cr-b_{20}RBC/SAv/b-Ab, non-injected, incubated with the antigen.

cause of the large circulation area contributed by the abundant lung capillaries. No specific accumulation of RBC label (^{51}Cr) in this organ is observed. The only organ that significantly removes immunoerythrocytes is spleen (Fig. 3). However, this clearance is not extensive and does not preclude the applicability of these modified erythrocytes.

The fate of the attached antibody matches that of the carrier cells (Fig. 3), with the only exception, already mentioned, of lungs. All this is also appreciated by analyzing the ratios between I and Cr isotopes (Fig 4) which are highest in the lung and somewhat increased in organs responsible for blood depuration, such as kidney or liver. Ratios in blood and heart are around 1, which confirms the permanence of b-Ab attached to the RBC.

All these data demonstrate the possibility to develop immunoerythrocytes that are stable in circulation. The question now is, "Do these immunoerythrocytes recognize the antigen, not only *in vitro* but also after their circulation *in vivo*?". The answer is offered in figure 5 where it is shown the recognition of the antigen (mouse IgG) by immunoerythrocytes (b_{20}RBC/SAv/b-Ab) both before and after having circulated. The recognition capacity of the two samples seems to be different, but this is due to the loss of b-Ab during the first minutes after the injection. The inset in Fig. 5 demonstrates the linear relationship between antigen (IgG) bound and antibody (b-Ab, anti-IgG) remaining attached to the RBC. This confirms the retention of the antigen binding capacity of immunoerythrocytes during circulation.

This work proves the possibility to develop immunoerythrocytes stable in the animal model and able to interact with the antigen. This may be a tool to deliver drug-carrier RBC to the target zone and to remove from the bloodstream harmful substances, virues, parasites, etc.

5. REFERENCES

1. E.A. Bayer and M. Wilchek, Protein biotinylation. Methods Enzymol. 184:138 (1990).
2. L. Chiarantini, R.E. Droleskey, M. Magnani, and J.R. DeLoach, In vitro targeting of erythrocytes to cytotoxic T-cells by coupling of Thy-1.2 monoclonal antibody. Biotechnol. Appl. Biochem. 15:171 (1992).
3. K. Kinosita and T.Y. Tsong, Voltage-induced pore formation and hemolysis of human erythrocytes. Nature 272:258 (1978).
4. D.L. Kooyman, G.W. Byrne, S. McClellan, D. Nielsen, M. Tone, H. Waldmann, T.M. Coffman, K.R. McCurry, J.L. Platt, and J.S. Logan, In vivo transfer of GPI-linked complement restriction factors from erythrocytes to the endothelium. Science 269:89 (1995).
5. M. Magnani, L. Chiarantini, E. Vittoria, U. Mancini, L. Rossi, and A. Fazi, Red blood cells as an antigen delivery system. Biotechnol. Appl. Biochem. 16:188 (1992).
6. V.R. Muzykantov and J.C. Murciano, Attachment of antibody to biotinylated red blood cells: Immunoerythrocytes display high affinity to immobilized antigen and normal biodistribution in rats. Biotechnol. Appl. Biochem. 24:41 (1996).
7. V.R. Muzykantov, J.C. Murciano, R.P. Taylor, E.N. Atochina, and A. Herráez, Regulation of the complement-mediated elimination of red blood cells modified with biotin and streptavidin. Anal. Biochem. 241:109 (1996).
8. V.R. Muzykantov, N. Seregina, and M. Smirnov, Fast lysis by complement and uptake by liver of avidin-carrying biotinylated erythrocytes. Int. J. Artif. Organs 15:622 (1992).
9. V.R. Muzykantov and R.P. Taylor, Attachment of biotinylated antibody to red blood cells: Antigen-binding capacity of immunoerythrocytes and their susceptibility to lysis by complement. Anal. Biochem. 223:142 (1994).
10. C. Ropars, B.P. Teisseire, M.C. Villereal, C. Bailleul, M. Chassaigne, and C. Nicolau, Engineered erythrocytes with high peripheral release of oxygen. In: "Biotechnology in Clinical Medicine", A. Albertini et al., eds. Raven Press, Ltd., New York (1987).
11. A.B. Zaltzman, K. van der Berg, V.R. Muzykantov, and B.P. Morgan, Enhanced complement susceptibility of avidin-biotin-treated human erythrocytes is a consequence of neutralization of the complement regulator CD59. Biochem. J. 307:651 (1995).

14

BIOCHEMICAL PROPERTIES OF ALCOHOL DEHYDROGENASE AND GLUTAMATE DEHYDROGENASE ENCAPSULATED INTO HUMAN ERYTHROCYTES BY A HYPOTONIC-DIALYSIS PROCEDURE

Silvia Sanz, Carmen Lizano, Marina I. Garín, José Luque, and Montserrat Pinilla

Dpto. Bioquimica y Biol. Mol.
Univ. Alcala
28871-Alcala de Henares
Madrid, Spain

1. SUMMARY

The stability against time (up to 170h) of encapsulated enzymes were studied in ADH- and GDH-carrier RBCs, at 4ºC and 37ºC, in comparison with that of free enzyme solutions. Encapsulation into RBCs suggest a protective effect of both enzyme activities. An efflux of the encapsulated enzymes from the carrier RBCs was observed during a similar incubation. The continuous degradation of ethanol and the simultaneous appearance/disappearance of acetaldehyde by ADH-RBCs, as a function of time (up to 72h), suggest the use of these carrier RBCs to fully metabolize ethanol. The rapid utilization of ammonia in the presence of GDH-RBCs suggest the use of these RBCs as carrier systems. These properties open the possibility of using ADH- and GDH-RBCs as carrier systems under *in vivo* situations.

2. INTRODUCTION

Human and animal red blood cells (RBCs) from different species can be engineered to behave as carriers of a wide variety of enzymes and other active proteins. Enzyme-loaded RBCs have been proposed in enzyme-replacement therapy as well as bioreactors for the enzymic degradation of plasma metabolites. The hypotonic-dialysis/isotonic-resealing procedure has been normally used for RBC encapsulation[2–6,8–11,13,16–19].

Erythrocytes as Drug Carriers in Medicine, edited by Sprandel and Way
Plenum Press, New York, 1997

The encapsulation of alcohol dehydrogenase (ADH; EC 1.1.1.1.) and glutamate dehydrogenase (GDH; EC 1.4.1.3.) in RBCs has been previously achieved in our laboratory[18]. While the yield of ADH-entrapment into human RBCs (17%) was not affected by the enzyme concentration in the dialysis bag, a significant increase in the yield of GDH-encapsulation (from 2% up to 36.2%) was found as the enzyme concentration was decreased (from 750U/mL down to 2U/mL RBC suspension; equivalent to 15–0.04mg enzyme protein/mL). The aggregation of GDH at protein levels above 1mg/mL[20] may explain not only the low GDH-encapsulation initially reported[2] but the inverse relationship between encapsulation and GDH concentration[18]. Therefore, both ADH-and GDH-RBCs can now be studied as potential carrier systems for the *in vivo* removal of ethanol and ammonia, respectively. The main goal of the present work is to show this metabolic capability *in vitro*. To this purpose, the stability with time of both encapsulated enzymes and their release from carrier-RBCs were also studied.

3. MATERIALS AND METHODS

3.1. RBC Suspensions and Erythrocyte Indexes

Human blood was drawn from healthy donors by venipuncture into heparinized tubes (10U/mL). The blood was centrifuged (1000xg, 10min, 4°C) and the plasma and buffy coat removed. RBCs were washed three times in isotonic Hanks-PBS (136.8mmol/L NaCl, 5.3mmol/L KCl, 0.43mmol/L Na_2HPO_4, 0.43mmol/L KH_2PO_4, 1.5mmol/L $MgCl_2$, 0.83mmol/L $MgSO_4$ and 6mmol/L glucose, pH 7.4). In the last wash the cell suspensions were centrifuged to obtain packed RBCs. RBC count (cells/L), hematocrit (Hct), mean cell volume (MCV), mean cell hemoglobin (MCH) and mean cell hemoglobin concentration (MCHC) were measured with an Hematology Analyzer System 9000 (Serono-Baker Diagnostic, Allentown, PA, USA).

3.2. Encapsulation of ADH and GDH and Determination of Enzyme Activities

Crystallized-lyophilized baker yeast ADH and bovine liver GDH were from Sigma-Aldrich Quimica, Spain. A hypotonic-dialysis/isotonic-resealing procedure was used[17,18]. Briefly, the packed RBCs (80–85% Hct) were mixed with the enzyme solutions and isotonic Hanks-PBS (70% Hct), and then dialysed (2–18/32" size bags; Medicell International Ltd) against 250mL of 40mOsm/Kg Hanks-PBS pH 7.4 (45min, 4ºC). The annealing step (10min at 37°C) was followed by cell resealing (30min at 37°C) in 1/10 (v/v) of modified (12% NaCl) PIGPA solution (100mmol/L pyruvate, 100mmol/L inosine, 100mmol/L glucose, 100mmol/L phosphate, 5mmol/L adenine), pH 7.4. RBCs were finally washed three times (800xg, 10min, 4°C) in Hanks-PBS, and resuspended in autologous plasma (1/3 v/v).

ADH activity was assayed according to Kennedy & Tipton[12]. GDH activity was assayed according to McCarty & Tipton[14]. The percentage of entrapped enzyme (encapsulation yield) is given by the enzyme activity within RBCs after the hypotonic/resealing process, referred to the initial enzyme activity of the RBC suspension added to the bag before dialysis (100%).

3.3. Ethanol, Acetaldehyde, and Ammonia Determinations

Ethanol and acetaldehyde concentration were determined by a gas chromatographic-headspace technique (Hewlett Packard 5890). The ammonia content was assayed by an enzymatic method (Boehringer Mannheim) as reported by Da Fonseca-Wollheim[1] .

4. RESULTS AND DISCUSSION

4.1. Encapsulation of ADH and GDH in Human RBCs

The encapsulation parameters are shown in Table I. These include cell recovery, encapsulation yield and erythrocytic indexes (MCV, MCH, MCHC) for the different RBC suspensions here used: native RBCs (Control), dialysed/resealed RBCs in the absence of enzymes (Control Unloaded) and dialysed/resealed RBCs in the presence of ADH or GDH (Loaded).

The percentage of cell recovery (61–72%) was rather high for the dialysed/resealed samples (i.e. unloaded, ADH-RBCs and GDH-RBCs). No apparent enzyme binding of ADH or GDH to native control RBCs (after incubation in the presence of enzymes) was observed (results not shown).

The encapsulation process was carried out at a fixed ADH or GDH level in the dialysis bag (50U/mL RBC suspension). Taking into account the specific activities of the commercial enzyme preparations, the 50 enzyme units are equivalent to 0.15mg ADH-protein and 1mg GDH-protein, respectively. The encapsulation yield for ADH (13%) and the low entrapment for GDH (1.9%) shown in Table I are in agreement with our previous work[18]. Such a low GDH-encapsulation is due to the relatively high enzyme protein concentration in the dialysis bag (1mg/mL) and the large extent of polymerization undergone by this hexameric enzyme at protein concentrations above 1mg/mL[20]. However, this low encapsulation yield is appropriate for the studies carried out in this paper. As previously reported[18], lower GDH concentrations in the dialysis bag (down to 0.04mg/mL) would give rise to higher encapsulation yields (up to 36.2%) but the specific activity would be so extremely low that these preparations seem to be not appropriated for either *in vitro* or *in vivo* studies.

Table 1. Encapsulation parameters and erythrocytic indexes (MCV, MCH and MCHC) for ADH- and GDH-RBCs. n=number of experiments (mean ±SEM)

		Dialysed/resealed RBCs		
			Encapsulation	
Parameter	Native RBCs	Control unloaded	ADH-RBCs	GDH-RBCs
n	5	6	6	6
Cell recovery (%)	97.8±0.8	61.8±2.2	72.4±3.3	63.2±2.8
Entrapment (%)	—	—	13±3.3	1.9±0.2
MCV (fl)	88.6±2.1	82.6±2.0	80.6±1.9	77.3±1.5
MCH (pg)	28.9±0.2	25.3±3.0	25.9±0.6	24.4±0.6
MCHC (g/dl)	32.8±0.8	30.7±0.6	32.3±1.0	31.7±1.2

As a consequence of the hypotonic dialysis procedure (Table I), a decrease in cell volume (MCV) from native (88.6 fL) to dialysed/resealed RBCs (77.3–82.6 fL) is observed. The decrease in hemoglobin content (MHC) from 28.9pg to 24.4–25.9pg is due to the loss of hemoglobin during encapsulation. These data are as previously reported for different carrier RBCs. Because of the smaller size (MCV) and the lower hemoglobin content (MCH) of carrier RBCs, the values of hemoglobin concentration (MCHC) are not significantly changed (Table I).

4.2. Stability of Encapsulated ADH and GDH

The stability of the enzymes in solution was compared with that of the entrapped enzymes under similar *in vitro* conditions. Free enzyme solutions (50U/mL) and suspensions of ADH- and GDH-loaded RBCs (25% Hct) were prepared in a modified Blood Bank CPDA solution formed by 1 volume of 327mg/mL citric acid, 2.63g/mL Na citrate, 2.92g/mL dextrose, 220mg/mL Na bisphosphate and 27mg/mL adenine plus 14 volumes of 150mmol/L NaCl and 1 volume of a commercial bactericide/fungicide solution (GIBCO-600–5240 PG). The mixtures were incubated (170 h, at 4°C or 37°C), and aliquots were taken at different times during the incubation to estimate ADH or GDH activities. The results are given as percentage of total enzyme activity at time zero.

As expected, at 4ºC, the activities of free ADH solutions (Fig 1A) and ADH-RBCs (Fig 1B) remain rather constant all along the time of incubation. However, at 37ºC, only

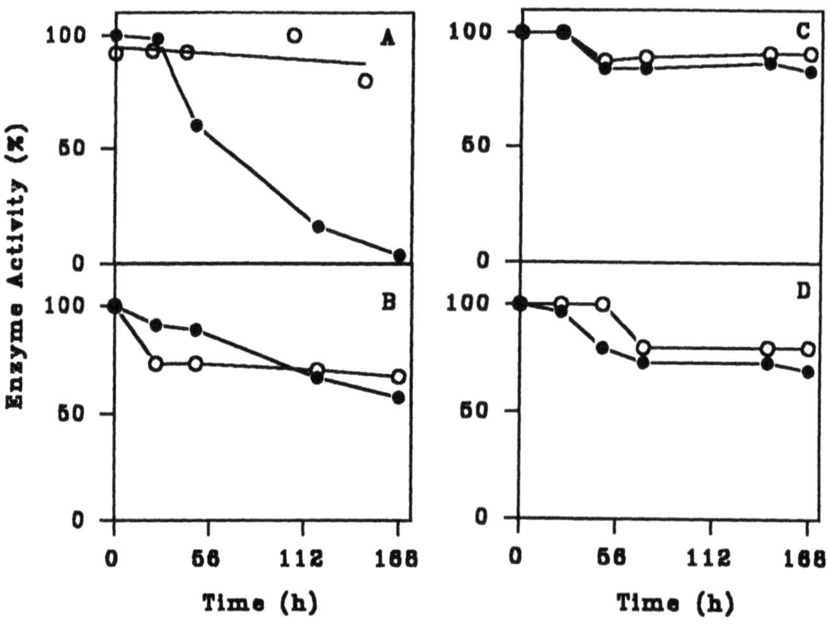

Figure 1. Stability of free ADH solution (A), ADH-RBC suspension (B), free GDH solution (C) and GDH-RBC suspension (D). Free enzyme solutions and enzyme-RBC suspensions (25% Hct) were prepared in a modificated CPDA medium (for details see 4.2. section) and incubated at 4°C (O) and 37°C (●) Values are mean of four experiments.

the activity of ADH solutions is significantly decreased (Fig 1A), probably because ADH denaturation with time. A slight decrease in activity is observed at 4ºC in ADH-RBCs (Fig 1B). Contrary to ADH, similar stability profiles were observed either at 4°C or 37°C for the free GDH solutions (Fig 1C) and the GDH-RBC preparations (Fig 1D). These results confirm that 4°C is an adequate temperature for both the free solutions and the encapsulated enzymes. They suggest that RBC encapsulation seems to exerts an adequate protective effect of the ADH activity at both 4ºC and the physiological temperature (37ºC). The hexameric character of GDH, which forms higher polymers at protein concentrations above 1 mg/mL[7,15] and the heat-stability of the bovine liver enzyme[20] (used in this work) may explain the stability at 37 ºC of the GDH solutions (Fig 1C). Because of the lack of aggregation of ADH, this protective effect was not observed at 37ºC in ADH solutions (Fig 1A).

In short, the stability with time of enzymes activity observed at 37ºC in ADH-RBCs (Fig1B) and GDH-RBCs (Fig 1D) indicate that RBC encapsulation seems to protect the activity of the loaded enzymes from premature degradation. This *in vitro* stability may be of significance from the point of view of the *in vivo* administration of enzyme-loaded RBCs

4.3. Release of ADH and GDH from Carrier RBCs

Fig 2 show the time course of total activity (in whole RBC suspensions) and released activity (in the supernatants) of ADH- and GDH-RBCs incubated at 4°C and 37°C during 170h in a CPDA solutions (25% Hct) (see Section 4.3). The results are given as percentage of enzyme activity at each time with respect to the activity at time zero of incubation.

The activity profiles for total ADH at 4ºC (Fig 2A) and 37ºC (Fig 2B), as well as those for GDH at 4ºC (Fig 2C) and 37ºC (Fig 2D) are quite similar to those shown in Fig 1.

The release of ADH and GDH was measured in the supernatants obtained after centrifugation (1000xg, 5min) of aliquots of the RBC suspensions taken at different times during the incubation. These supernatants contain an accumulative amount of the free enzymes released to the medium at each specific time. The data in Fig 2 about release of enzymes are not affected by any cellular breakdown, as indicated by the constant number of total RBCs (autoanalyzer cell counting; results not shown) during the whole period of incubation. As shown in Fig 2, during the first 24 hr of incubation, no release of ADH was observed at 4ºC (Fig 2A) or 37ºC (Fig 2B). Then, the activity in the supernatant increased with time at both temperatures. It should means that the membrane pores formed during the hypotonic treatment, which still remain as smaller residual pores after the resealing step, allow the efflux of the entrapped proteins from carrier RBCs[21]. Such a release is more pronounced at 4°C (Fig 2A) than 37°C (Fig 2B), thus indicating that the lower temperature (4ºC) may be either affecting the releasing process and/or the activity of the released ADH in the supernatant. The latter assumption is in agreement with data shown in Fig 1A, in which a significant protective effect of the activity of ADH in solution was observed at 4ºC but not at 37ºC.

Figure 2 also show the changes in the released GDH. At 4°C (Fig 2C), no GDH activity was observed in the supernatants during the first 62 h of incubation. Then, the activity slightly increases with time. At 37°C (Fig 2D), the activity of released GDH is clearly observed in the supernatant from time zero, to reach a constant rising value up to 170 h. This could be an indication of a sustained release of the encapsulated GDH at 37ºC. This

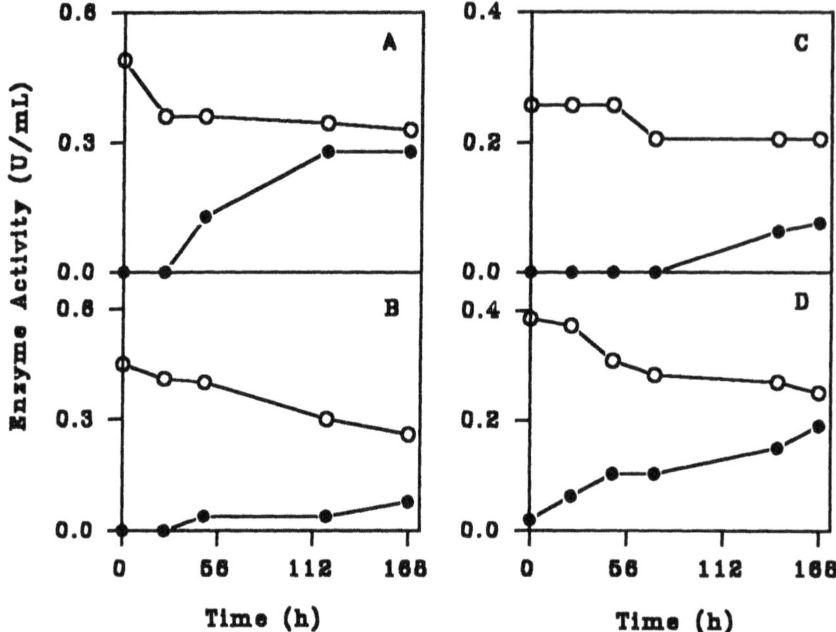

Figure 2. *In vitro* ADH released at 4°C (A) and 37°C (B) and GDH released at 4°C (C) and 37°C (D) from carrier RBCs. These suspensions were prepared at 25% Hct in a modificated CPDA medium. The total ADH and GDH activities were measured in the whole ADH- and GDH-RBC suspensions (○). The released ADH and GDH activities were measured in their respective supernatants (●). The values for ADH and GDH activities remaining within loaded-RBCs (□) were those given by the difference between total and released enzymes. Values are the mean of three experiments.

is supported by data on heat-stability of the bovine liver enzyme[20] as well as on the stability results shown for GDH solutions at 37ºC (Fig 1C).

4.4. Metabolic Properties of ADH- and GDH-RBCs

In this section, the *in vitro* metabolic capability of ADH and GDH-RBCs (i.e. the catalytic effect on their respective enzyme reactions) was studied. This is an essential prerequisite for its potential use as *in vivo* carrier enzyme systems to eliminate high blood levels of ethanol and ammonia, respectively.

4.4.1. Ethanol Degradation and Acetaldehyde Formation. ADH-RBCs were suspended in Hanks-PBS (30% Hct) and ethanol was added as substrate (0.1%; 30mmol/L). The cellular suspensions, as well as native RBCs as a control, were transferred into 10mL vial and then sealed. The vials are then incubated at 37°C for 170h. At different times, two vials (sample and control) were taken and frozen at -80°C until direct evaluation of ethanol and acetaldehyde by gas chromatography.

As shown in Figure 3A, the level of initial ethanol (30mmol/L) is not affected by the incubation with native RBCs. However, ADH-RBCs continuously degrade it. For instance, 70% (21mmol/L) and 30% (9mmol/L) of the initial ethanol remain at 15–17h and

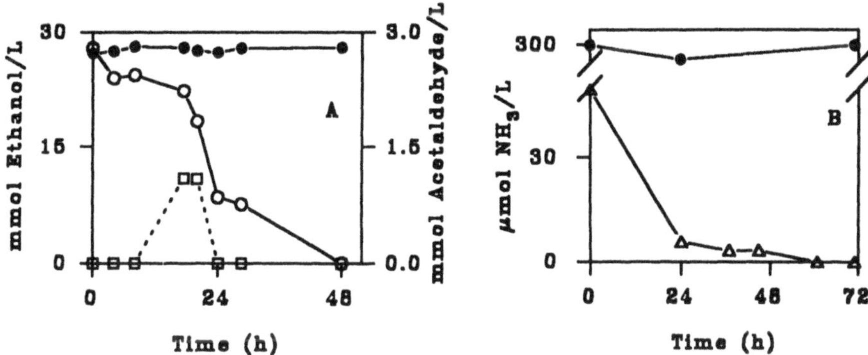

Figure 3. *In vitro* ethanol (O) and acetaldehyde (□) degradation by ADH-loaded RBCs (A), and ammonia (Δ) utilization by GDH-loaded RBCs (B). Native RBC suspensions (●). For details see 4.4.1. section. Values are the mean of three different experiments.

24h, respectively, to totally disappear at 48h. On the other hand, an appearance/disappearance peak of acetaldehyde is observed at a time (15–17h) during the 48h period of continuous ethanol degradation. Both observations may be explained on the basis of: a) the encapsulated ADH, which degrade ethanol to acetaldehyde; and b) the presence in native RBCs of the cytosolic high-Km form of acetaldehyde dehydrogenase (EC 1.2.1.3; ALDH)[22], which degrade acetaldehyde to acetate. From these results, it can be suggested for our ADH-RBCs to be able to simultaneously degrade ethanol and acetaldehyde.

4.4.2. Ammonia Utilization. GDH-loaded RBCs were suspended in Hanks-PBS (30% Hct) containing 300µmol/L NH_4Cl and 13mmol/L α-ketoglutarate as substrates. The cellular suspensions and the native RBCs were incubated at 37°C during 72h, and aliquots were withdraw at different times and centrifuged (1000xg 5min). The supernatants were kept frozen (-80°C) until use.

As shown in Figure 3B, the level of initial ammonia (300µmol/L) is not affected during the incubation with native RBCs. However, GDH-RBCs rapidly use ammonia. For instance, only 5% (15µmol/L) of the initial ammonia remains at 24h of incubation. These results clearly suggest that the encapsulation of bovine liver GDH in human RBCs might be appropriated for the removal of high levels of ammonia in blood.

5. REFERENCES

1. Da Fonseca-Wollheim, F. (1973) The significance of the hydrogen ion concentration and the addition of ADP in the determination of ammonia with glutamate dehydrogenase: An improved enzyme determination of ammonia *J. Clin. Chem. Clin. Biochem.* **11,** 421–426
2. De Flora, A. (1985). The technology of carrier erythrocytes: a versatile tool for diagnosis and therapy. In: *Biotechnology in Diagnostics,*(Koprowski H, Ferrone S, Albertini A Eds.) Elsevier Science Publishers B.V. (Biomedical Division) 223–236
3. DeLoach, J.R. (1986). Carrier erythrocytes. *Med Res Rev* **6,** 487–504
4. DeLoach, J.R. (1987). Dialysis method for entrapment of proteins into resealed red blood cells. *Methods Enzymol* **149,** 235–242

5. DeLoach, J.R. and Sprandel, U. Eds. (1985) *Red blood Cells and Carriers for Drugs*. Krenger, Basilea
6. DeLoach, J.R. and Way, J.L. Eds. (1994). Carrier and bioreactor red blood cells for drug delivery and targeting. *Advances in the Biosciences* **92,** Pergamon, Great Britain
7. Eisenberg, H., Josephs, R. and Reisler, E. (1976) Bovine liver glutamate dehydrogenase. *Adv Protein Chem* **30,** 101
8. Fazi, A., Mancini, U., Mangani, F., Accorsi, A., Piatti, E., Rossi, L .and Magnani, M. (1994) *In vitro* and *in vivo* methanol degradation by alcohol oxidase-loaded erythrocytes *Advances in the Biosciences* **92,** 93–100
9. Garín, M., Rossi, L., Luque, J. and Magnani, M. (1995) Lactate catabolism by enzyme-loaded red blood cells *Biotechnol. Appl. Biochem* **22,** 295–303
10. Garín,M., López,R., Sanz,S., Pinilla,M. and Luque,J. (1996). Erythrocytes as carriers for recombinant human erythropoietin. *Pharm.Res.* **13,** 869–874
11. Ihler, G.M. (1983) Erythrocyte carriers *Pharmac. Ther.* **20,** 151–169
12. Kennedy, N.P. and Tipton, K.F. (1990) Ethanol metabolism and alcoholic liver disease. *Assays in Biochemistry* **25,** 137–195
13. Magnani, M. and DeLoach, J.R. Eds. (1992) The Use of Resealed Erythrocytes as Carriers and Bioreactors. *Adv. Exp. Med. Biol.* **326,** Plenum Press, New York
14. McCarty, A.D. and Tipton, K.F. (1985) Ox glutamate dehydrogenase comparison of the kinetic properties of native and proteolysed preparation *Biochem J* **230,** 95
15. Reisler, E., Pouyet, J. and Eisenberg, H. (1970). Molecular weights, association, and frictional resistance of bovine liver glutamate dehydrogenase at low concentrations. Equilibrium and velocity sedimentation, light-scattering studies, and settling experiments with macroscopic models of the enzyme oligomer. *Biochemistry* **9,**:3095.
16. Ropars, C., Chassaigne, M. and Nicolau, C. Eds. (1987) *Red blood cells as a carrier for drug* Pergamon, Oxford
17. Ropars, C., Chassaigne, M., Villereal, M.C., Avenard, G., Hurel, C. and Nicolau, C. (1985) Resealed red blood cells as a new blood transfusion product *Biblthca Haemat* **51,** 82–91
18. Sanz, S., Pinilla, M., Garín, M., Tipton, K.F. and Luque, J. (1995) The influence of enzyme concentration on the encapsulation of glutamate dehydrogenase and alcohol dehydrogenase in red blood cells *Biotechnol. Appl. Biochem* **22,** 223–231
19. Sprandel, U. (1994) Erythrocytes as carriers of therapeutic enzymes in inherited metabolic diseases *Advances in the Biosciences* **92,** 191–198.
20. Tipton, K.F. and Couee, I. (1988) Glutamate Dehydrogenase In: *Glutamine and Glutamate in Mammals.* (G. Kuamme, Ed.). CRC Press. Boca Raton, Florida, pp. 81–100
21. Zolla, L., Lupidi, G., Marcheggiani, M., Falcioni, G. and Brunori, M. (1990) Encapsulation of proteins into human erythrocytes: a kinetic investigation *Biochim. Biophys. Acta* **1024,** 5–9
22. Zorzano, A. and Herrera, E. (1990) Differences in the kinetic properties and sensitivity to inhibitors of human placental, erythrocyte, and major hepatic aldehyde dehydrogenase isoenzymes *Biochem Pharmacol* **39,** 873–878

INFLUENCE OF CHEMICAL MODIFICATION ON "*IN VIVO*" AND "*IN VITRO*" MOUSE CARRIER ERYTHROCYTE SURVIVAL AND RECOGNITION

J. A. Jordán,[1] F. J. Alvarez,[1] J. C. Murciano,[1] A. Lotero,[1] A. Herráez,[1] M. C. Tejedor,[1] J. Luque,[1] J. R. DeLoach,[2] and J. C. Díez[1]

[1]Departamento de Bioquímica y Biología Molecular
Campus Universitario
Universidad de Alcalá
28871 Alcalá de Henares
Madrid, Spain
[2]USDA.ARS-FAPL
College Station, Texas 77845

1. INTRODUCTION

Several systems have been developed with therapeutical purposes for drug delivery. Among them, red blood cells (RBCs) have been claimed to be a physiological method to convey and deliver active compounds.[4,6,8,11] The preparation of erythrocytes as carriers can require encapsulation procedures or/and chemical modification of erythrocyte surface.[3,22] In fact, the efficacy of these systems can be dependent of the use of several chemical treatments which can react with cell membrane proteins. Crosslinking reagents can be applied to red blood cell modification. Glutaraldehyde (GA) has been the most extensively used crosslinker.[7,21] Also, other crosslinkers can be applied to carrier erythrocytes preparation.[12,16] Biotinylation is another alternative method for carrier preparation.[15,19] Eventually, chemical modification can promote targeting of carrier erythrocytes to several organs.[12,21] We have focused our attention on the action of crosslinking reagents which react with band 3 in mouse erythrocyte membrane. Additionally, biotinylation of mouse erythrocytes has been studied. "*In vivo*" behaviour of these chemically modified erythrocytes have been studied. These survival results have been compared to recognition by macrophages. Thus, we described conditions for using these chemical treatments for targeting to organs and macrophages.

Erythrocytes as Drug Carriers in Medicine, edited by Sprandel and Way
Plenum Press, New York, 1997

2. MATERIALS AND METHODS

2.1. Materials

Bis(Sulfosuccinimidyl)Suberate (BS^3) and 3,3′-Dithiobis(Sulfosuccinimidylpropionate) (DTSSP) were supplied by Pierce Rockford, IL, USA. N-Hydroxysuccinimide Ester of Biotin (NHS-X-Biotin) and Streptavidin (SAv) was obtained from calbiochem. ATP and Glutathione (GSH) were from Boehringer (Boehringer, Mannheim, Germany). the dialysis bag was from Medicell (Medicell, London, UK). Other chemicals used were reagent grade and were purchased from Merck (Merck, Darmstad, Germany)

2.2. Animals

CD1 mice weighing 25 g (6–8 weeks old) were used in this study. They were kept at controlled conditions of temperature and humidity, with day-night cycles according to European Union directives.

2.3. Isolation of Erythrocytes

Erythrocytes suspensions were prepared from CD1 mouse whole blood. Plasma, white blood cells and platelets were separated by centrifugation (500 x g for 10 min. at 4° C). Erythrocyte pellets were washed three times in saline phosphate buffer (PBS) solution containing either 145 mM NaCl, 5 mM glucose, 5 mM K_2HPO_4/NaH_2PO_4 pH 7.4 for biotinylated and crosslinked erythrocytes or 9 mM glucose, 4 mM $MgCl_2$, 5 mM inosine, 5 mM Adenosine, 21,5 mM K_2HPO_4/NaH_2PO_4 pH 7.4 for hypotonically treated and crosslinked erythrocytes and centrifuged as above. Last centrifugation was carried out at 2 500 x g for 10 min for samples used for hypotonic dialysis. The final erythrocyte pellet (Haematocrit 90%) were used for encapsulation treatments.

2.4. Cell Counting and Cell Size Determination

These two parameters were determined in a Hematology Analyzer (Serono-Baker diagnostics System 2000 Plus).

2.5. Encapsulation Procedure

Hypotonic treatments for marker proteins encapsulation was done using dialysis medium previously described.[12] Washing media used were those indicated previously. [1,5]

2.6. Chemical crosslinking of Erythrocytes

Treatments with BS^3 and DTSSP were accomplished as described.[17,18] Crosslinking of mouse erythrocytes with bifunctional reagents was carried out by adding erythrocytes ($1.7x10^9$ cell/ml in phosphate buffer containing 5 mM glucose, 106 mM Na_2HPO_4/NaH_2PO_4 pH 7.4) to BS^3 or DTSSP in 53 mM phosphate buffer in a 1:1 ratio, followed by an incubation for 30 minutes at room temperature with gentle agitation. The final concentration of bifunctional reagent was 5 mM. The reaction was stopped by adding approximately 20 volumes of 0.15 M NaCl, 25 mM Tris pH 7.4 buffer.

2.7. Biotinylation of RBCs and Quantitation of Its Residues with Radiolabelled SAv

The biotinylation procedure was performed as described.[15] Briefly, RBCs were obtained from heparinized mouse blood by four washes with PBS-saline (pH 7.6). 1 ml of 10% suspension of washed RBC in PBS was supplemented with 100 μl of 0.3 M of borate buffer saline (pH 9.0) and 7 μl of 0.1 M N-hidroxy-sulccinimide ester of Biotin(NHS-X-Biotin) solution in dimethylformamide. After 30 minutes of incubation at room temperature, cells were washed three times in PBS-Bovine Serum Albumin (BSA) (1 mg/ml) and resuspended in the same buffer. 10 μl of biotinylated erythrocytes were resuspended in 100 μl of native RBCs and 4 μl of a 0.25 mg/ml solution of radiolabelled-SAv (10^6 molecules/RBC) in saline were added to the RBC suspension. After 20 minutes of incubation at room temperature, unbound SAv was removed by washing 3 times with PBS-BSA (1 mg/ml). Cells were resuspended and counted in a gamma-counter.

2.8. Isolation of Membranes

Erythrocyte membrane isolation was performed as described previously.[17,18]

2.9. Electrophoretic Analyses and Densitometric Scanning

Analytical SDS-polyacrylamide gel electrophoresis was performed as described.[10] ß-mercaptoethanol was avoided in the case of DTSSP-crosslinked mouse erythrocyte membranes in order to prevent disruption of crosslinker structure by reducing reagents. For densitometric scanning of the gels, a LKB Ultroscan XL Densitometer, with Gelscan XL programme, was used. Erythrocyte membranes from mouse untreated and crosslinked erythrocytes were run on SDS-polyacrylamide gel electrophoresis. To analyze the crosslinking of band 3 protein, it was measured the proportion of band 3 monomer present in the densitometric scans of membranes from untreated erythrocytes with respect to the total membrane proteins present in the gels by integration of the area under the peaks. This value correspond to the percentage of band 3 protein monomer in relation to the whole protein present in the untreated sample (a). Similarly, it was calculated the proportion of band 3 monomer present in the densitometric scans of membranes from crosslinked erythrocytes with respect to the total membrane proteins present in the gels by integration of the area under the peaks. This value correspond to the percentage of band 3 protein monomer in relation to the whole protein present in the crosslinked sample (b). This second value (b) was always lower than the first one (a). From these two values, it can be calculated the reduction of the proportion of band 3 protein monomer in the crosslinked samples. (b/a) x 100 gives the percentage of band 3 protein monomer which remains uncrosslinked after the crosslinking treatment. 100 - [(b/a) x 100] could be used as a value for estimation of the extent of crosslinking.

2.10. Radioactive Labeling

Chromium labeling of erythrocytes was done with chromium (^{51}Cr) by mixing 100 μl $Na_2{}^{51}CrO_4$ in isotonic saline (1.0 mCi/ml, Dupont NEN, Brussels, Belgium) with one milliliter of erythrocytes (10^{10} cells/ml) SAv radiolabelling was performed by the Iodogen procedure (Pierce) according to the manufacturer's recommendations.

2.11. *In Vivo* Survival of Modified Erythrocytes

For *in vivo* experiments, ^{51}Cr-erythrocytes were crosslinked as described above using a crosslinker concentration of 5 mM. ATP 0.25 mM and reduced glutathione (GSH) 0.5 mM were added to the solutions used in cell isolation, labeling and washing, in order to prevent cell oxidation processes. The labeled erythocytes were washed 2 times in PBS and resuspended to around 10^{10} erythrocytes/ml for experimental use. Mice were injected with 100 μl of control (untreated cells which were incubated in the same medium but in the absence of chemical reagent) or modified ^{51}Cr-erythrocytes intraperitoneally (i.p.)in the case of crosslinked erythrocytes and intravenously in the case of biotinylated erythrocytes. At time zero (within 10 minutes after injection) and at different times after injection from 3 to 10 mice of each group were bled and liver, spleen, lungs and kidneys taken. The radioactivity present in the organs and 10 μl of blood was determined using a LKB-Wallac 1282 compugamma CS counter.

Injection of biotinylated RBCs in mice, "*in vivo*" behaviour analysis and biodistribution study were done as follows. CD1 mice were anesthetized with i.p. injection of sodium pentobarbital solution (50 mg/kg). 20 μl of a 10% suspension of biotinylated RBCs radiolabelled with $^{51}CrO_4Na$, as previously described, were mixed with 200 μl of native RBC. This suspension was injected by the tail vein. 200 μl of blood were collected from the eye. At 1 hour after injection, animals were killed, blood and internal organs were collected. Organs were also rinsed in saline to remove blood. Levels of ^{51}Cr were measured in a gamma-counter.

2.12. Macrophage Recognition Assays

Preparation of peritoneal macrophages were prepared as described.[13] Adhesion and phagocitosis assays for erythrocyte recognition by macrophages were done as indicated.[20]

3. RESULTS

3.1. Extent of Modification

First, we evaluated the extent of crosslinking and biotinylation produced in mouse erythrocytes (Table 1). The action of these reagents on band 3 can be observed by analysis of erythrocyte membranes by SDS-PAGE. Bands of higher molecular weight and high molecular weight precipitates are produced as a result of the chemical reaction. The reduction of the proportion of band 3 monomer in electrophoretic gels can be used as an estimation of the crosslinking of band 3. Mouse native erythrocytes were crosslinked with BS^3 and DTSSP. At 5 mM, BS^3 and DTSSP rendered around 28–29% of Band 3 crosslinking in mouse erythrocyte membranes. Slightly lower crosslinking can be observed in the case of mouse erythrocytes which were previously treated by hypotonic dialysis for protein encapsulation. The extent of band 3 crosslinking seemed to be lower when DTSSP was used in comparison to crosslinking with BS^3.

Additionally, the levels of biotinylation raised in mouse erythrocytes were evaluated. In the conditions described in Methods, biotinylation levels accounted for 6 x 10^5 molecules of bound Streptavidin per cell (see also Table 1).

Table 1. Extent of the chemical modification in mouse erythrocytes. Extent of chemical crosslinking was estimated as level of band 3 monomer which were crosslinked in higher molecular weight oligomers. Biotinylation levels were estimated by measuring the number of streptavidin molecules bound per mouse erythrocyte

	Chemical treatment		
Modified Cell type	BS^3 5mM (% Band 3 reduction)	DTSSP 5mM (% Band 3 reduction)	NHS-BIOTIN (SAv molecules/RBC)
Native RBCs	29.30	28.10	6.4×10^5
Loaded RBCs	21.13	17.54	

3.2. *In Vivo* Survival and Organ Localization of Biotinylated RBC

As it can be observed in Fig. 1, biotinylated erythrocytes did not circulate since extremely low levels of radioactivity corresponding to labelled biotinylated erythrocytes can be observed in blood. Biotinylated erythrocytes are uptaken by liver since at 1 hour after injection around 30% of the total injected radioactivity is recovered by this organ. At this time, almost no biotinylated erythrocytes was observed in circulation. Other organs showed also recovered radioactivity, although the level of chromium present in these organs are very low (Fig.1).

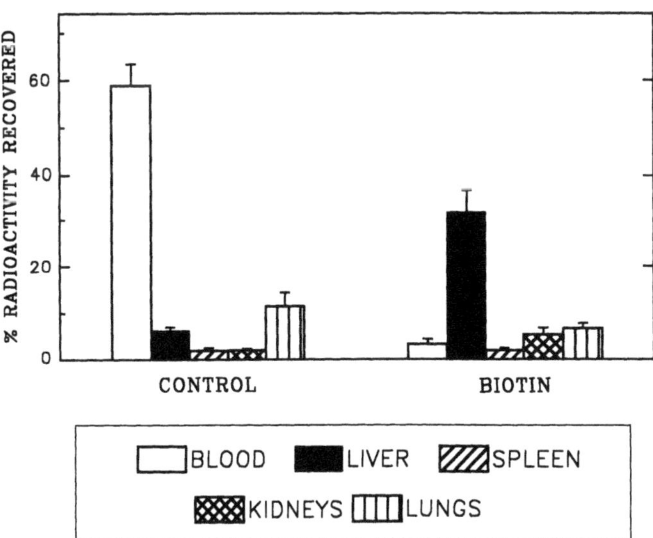

Figure 1. "*In vivo*" survival and radioactivity localization of biotinylated erythrocytes in different organs. This figure shows a diagramatic scheme showing the percentages of radioactivity present in different organs at 1 hour times after injection of labeled erythrocytes. The percentage of radioactivity from labeled erythrocytes collected in blood and in different organs is shown. The percentages represent absolute values in relation to the total injected radioactivity. The values correspond to the mean value ± S.E.M. From 3 to 10 animals were used.

3.3. *In Vivo* Survival and Organ Localization of Crosslinked Erythrocytes

We have also analyzed the survival of mouse erythrocytes which were incubated with crosslinkers which react with band 3 protein in erythrocyte membrane. Crosslinking with both reagents (BS^3 and DTSSP) rendered erythrocytes which after injection into mouse are predominantly targeted to liver (Fig. 2). Spleen also showed a significant recovery of chromium radioactivity. As it can be observed, only a slight increase in the percentage of recovered radioactivity in liver can be observed as a function of the time, since very similar values were obtained at 4 h. and 24 h. for the two crosslinkers studied.

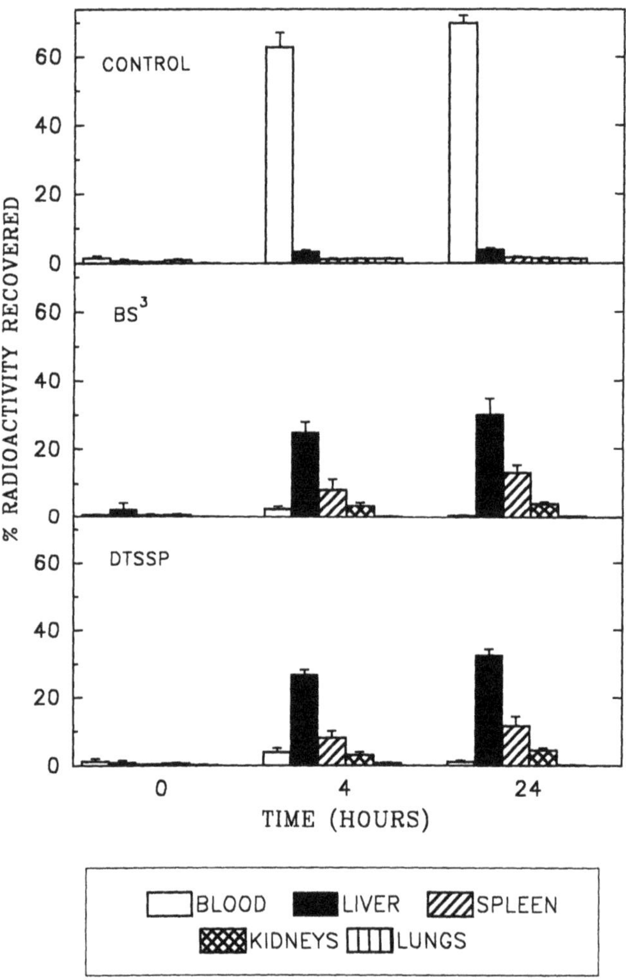

Figure 2. "*In vivo*" survival and radioactivity localization of crosslinked erythrocytes in different organs (Crosslinker concentration 5 mM). This figure shows a diagramatic scheme showing the percentages of radioactivy present in blood and in different organs at different times after injection of labeled erythrocytes. The percentage of radioactivity from labeled erythrocytes collected in blood and in different organs is shown. The percentages represent absolute values in relation to the total injected radioactivity. The values correspond to the mean value ± S.E.M.. From 3 to 10 animals were used.

3.4. *In Vivo* Survival and Organ Localization of Crosslinked Loaded Erythrocytes

Preparation of carrier erythrocytes can involve hypotonic dialysis incorporation of active compounds and subsequent modification of erythrocyte membrane with different purposes such as obtaining an increase in cell stability, producing targeting of the loaded erythrocytes, etc. Thus, we analyzed the behaviour of erythrocytes, which having been treated by hypotonic shock, were subsequently treated with crosslinking reagents (Fig. 3).

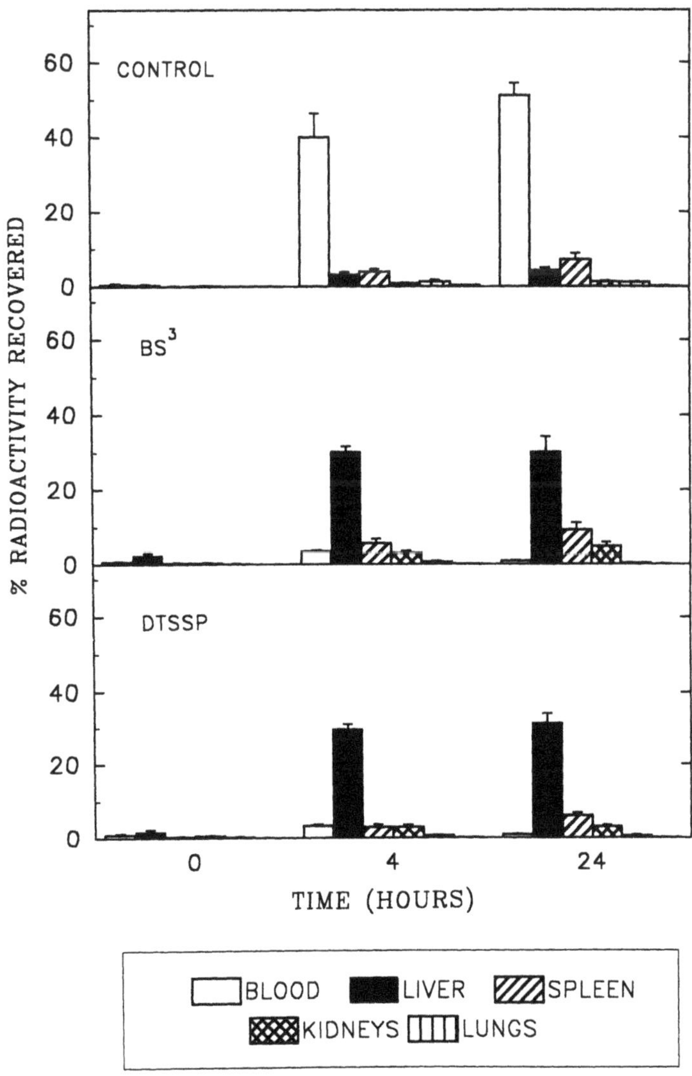

Figure 3. "*In vivo*" survival and radioactivity localization of crosslinked hypotonically treated erythrocytes in different organs (Crosslinker concentration 5 mM). This figure shows a diagrammatic scheme showing the percentages of radioactivity present in blood and in different organs at different times after injection of labeled erythrocytes. The percentage of radioactivity from labeled erythrocytes collected in blood and in different organs is shown. The percentages represent absolute values in relation to the total injected radioactivity. The values correspond to the mean value ± S.E.M. From 3 to 10 animals were used.

Crosslinked and hypotonically treated erythrocytes revealed a similar behaviour to crosslinked erythrocytes. These treatments also gave rise to a predominant recognition by liver, although also in this case a small level of radioactivity can be found in spleen. As it is shown in Fig. 3 slightly higher values of radioactivity present in liver was observed at 24 h. in comparison to the results obtained for 4 h. analyses. Also, similar patterns were obtained for BS^3 and DTSSP crosslinked erythrocytes. Additionally, the obtained values for these modified erythrocytes were similar to those found for erythrocytes which were only crosslinked (Fig. 2 and Fig. 3).

3.5. Macrophage Recognition of Modified Erythrocytes

In order to correlate "*in vivo*" targeting to organs of modified erythrocytes with "*in vitro*" behaviour of these cells, we have studied the interaction between chemically treated erythrocytes and macrophages obtained from mouse peritoneal cavity. Macrophage recognition studies showed a close relationship with "*in vivo*" studies. Biotinylated erythrocytes are highly recognized by peritoneal macrophages since around 50% of total radioactivity present in erythrocytes seemed to be present in plates analyzed for macrophage recognition. Native and hypotonically treated erythrocytes showed similar values of macrophages recognition in the conditions used (5–8% of radioactivity present in labelled erythrocytes). In contrast crosslinked erythrocytes are recognized by peritoneal macrophages in a significant higher proportion (around 70% for BS^3 crosslinked erythrocytes and 50% for DTSSP treated erythrocytes). When hypotonic dialysis was carried out previously to crosslinking treatments, these modified erythrocytes are less recognized than erythrocytes which were only crosslinked.

4. DISCUSSION

Carrier targeting has been stablished as an appropriate way to increase action efficiency in drug delivery systems.[12,21] Different methods can be used to target carrier erythrocytes. Chemical modification by crosslinkers has been used to target erythrocytes on which ß-galactosidase,[20] methotrexate,[7] adriamycin,[21] etc. were previously loaded. Some chemical crosslinkers such glutaraldehyde (GA) react extensively with a variety of proteins in erythrocyte membrane.[7,20,21] In these cases, quantitation of the membrane modification may result difficult to determine. Chemical crosslinking of specific proteins in erythrocyte membrane can be accomplished.[17,18] Band 3 protein is crosslinked when erythrocytes from different species are incubated with reagents such as BS^3 and DTSSP.[2,9,17,18] Quantitative determination of the action of these two reagents on band 3 protein can be carried out (See methods). Crosslinking of mouse erythrocyte band 3 accounted for values ranging around 28–29% (Table 1), what is significantly lower than for its human counterpart.[17,18] Furthermore, the described conditions for mouse erythrocyte band 3 crosslinking can be applied to hypotonically treated mouse erythrocytes. Lower extent of band 3 crosslinking might be a consequence of the hypotonic shock to what these cells were subjected. Anyhow, the level of band 3 crosslinking in mouse hypotonically treated erythrocytes is not much lower than in the case of untreated erythrocytes what revealed that the crosslinker is acting in a similar way on both types of cells (Table 1). Erythrocyte biotinylation has been previously described. In this work, quantitative determination by measuring bound Streptavidin molecules showed a high level of biotinylation of mouse erythrocytes (see also Table 1).[15]

Biotinylation conditions described here allowed recovery of modified labelled erythrocytes in liver, what make them useful for targeting application. "*In vivo*" behaviour of chemically modified erythrocytes showed preferential targeting to liver. Band 3 crosslinked erythrocytes when injected into animals were localized in liver, although some deposition in spleen was also observed (Fig.2). The radioactivity recovery at 4 h. and 24 h. after intraperitoneal injection were very similar. Thus, 5 mM band 3 crosslinker concentration is adequate for targeting of mouse erythrocytes. This is the case for the two reagents used, BS^3 and DTSSP. Preparation of carrier erythrocytes usually requires encapsulation procedures involving hypotonic shock for incorporation of active compounds.[3,8,22] Crosslinking of loaded erythrocytes can render targeted carrier cells.[7,12,21] Crosslinking by BS^3 and DTSSP of erythrocytes treated for encapsulation was also studied by "*in vivo*" experiments. The conditions described in the present work gave rise to predominant localization of labelling in liver after injection of chromium labelled erythrocytes (Fig.3). Similar levels of radioactivity localized in liver were observed in these carrier erythrocytes in comparison to crosslinked erythrocytes. This might be explained considering the similar extent of band 3 crosslinking which can be observed in hypotonically treated erythrocytes crosslinked with BS^3 and DTSSP (see Table 1) in comparison to only crosslinked erythrocytes. Thus, band 3 oligomerization as a consequence of crosslinking can be the cause of mouse erythrocytes targeting. Nevertheless, release of intracellular chromium labelling as a result of an increased fragility of hypotonically treated erythrocytes with respect to native erythrocytes might also be considered.[14] These results are similar to those described by other authors who use band 3 clustering to produce erythrocyte targeting.[2]

"*In vitro*" analyses for macrophages recognition of erythrocytes treated in the experimental conditions here described showed a close relationship to the survival in circulation results. This indicates the feasibility of the conditions used to assess the chemical modification produced in mouse erythrocytes. Additionally, these conditions can be used for "*in vivo*" targeting and also for studying carrier erythrocyte-macrophage interaction.

5. ACKNOWLEDGMENTS

This work was supported in part by grants from D.G.I.C.y T. (PB92/0172 and PB94/0367), C.I.C. y T. (FAR 90/102), F.I.S. (93/1040) and U.A.H (032/96). J.A. Jordán is a recipient of fellowships from Universidad de Alcalá de Henares and Comunidad Autónoma de Madrid. F.J.Alvarez was also supported by fellowships from Universidad de Alcalá de Henares and Comunidad Autónoma de Madrid. A. Lotero is a fellow from Glaxo-U.A.H.

6. REFERENCES

1. L. Chiarantini, J. Johnson and J. R. DeLoach, Optimized recirculation survival of mouse carrier erythrocytes, Blood Cells 17:607 (1991)
2. L. Chiarantini, L. Rossi, A. Fraternale and M. Magnani, Modulated red blood cell survival by membrane protein clustering, Mol. Cell Biochem. 144:53 (1995)
3. J.R.DeLoach, Encapsulation of exogenous agents and the circulating survival of carrier erythrocytes, J.Appl. Biochem. 5:149 (1983)
4. J.R. DeLoach, Carrier erythrocytes, Med. Res. Rev. 6:487 (1986).

5. J.R. DeLoach and R. Drosleskey, Survival of murine carrier erythrocytes injected via peritoneum, Comp. Biochem. Physiol. 84A:447 (1986)
6. J.R.DeLoach and U. Sprandel, Eds, Red Blood Cells as Carriers for Drugs, Karger, Basel (1985)
7. J.R.DeLoach, C.H. Tangner and C. Barton, Hepatic pharmacokinetics of glutaraldehyde-treated methrotrexate-loaded carrier erythrocytes in dogs, Res. Exp. Med. 183, 167 (1983)
8. G.M. Ihler, Erythrocyte Carriers, Pharmac. Ther. 20:151 (1983)
9. J.A. Jordán, J.R. DeLoach, J. Luque and J.C. Díez, Targeting of mouse erythrocytes by band 3 crosslinkers, Biochim. Biophys. Acta. 1291:27 (1996).
10. U.K.Laemmli, Cleavage of structural proteins during the assembly of the head of bacteriophage T4, Nature 227:680 (1970)
11. M. Magnani and J. R. DeLoach,Eds, The Use of Resealed Erythrocytes as Carriers and Bioreactors,Plenum Press, New York (1992)
12. M.Magnani, L. Rossi, G. Brandi, G.F. Schiavano, M. Montroni and G. Piedimonte, Targeting antiretroviral nucleoside analogues in phosphorylated form to macrophages: *In vitro* and *in vivo* studies, Proc. Natl. Acad. Sci. USA, 89:6477 (1992)
13. M.S. Meltzer, Peritoneal mononuclear phagocytes from small animals in Methods for studying mononuclear phagocytes. D.O. Adams; P.J. Edelson and H. Koren, eds. Academic Press pp. 63–67 (1981)
14. M. Morrison, A.W. Michaels, D.R. Phillips and S. Choi. Life span of erythrocyte membrane protein, Nature 248:763 (1974)
15. V. Muzykantov and R. Taylor, Attachment of biotinylated antibody to red blood cells: Antigen binding capacity of immunoerythrocytes and their susceptibility to lysis by complement, Anal. Biochem. 223:142 (1994)
16. M. Pinilla, J. Luque, and K. Tipton, Modification in the allosteric properties of phosphofructokinase in rat erythrocyte and reticulocyes cross-linked with dimethylsuberimidate and 3,3′-dithiobispropionimidate, Biochim. Biophys. Acta 702:254 (1982)
17. J.V. Staros, N-hydroxysulfosuccinimide active esters: Bis(N-hydroxysulfosuccinimide) esters of dicarboxylic acids are hydrophilic membrane-impermeant, protein cross-linkers, Biochemistry 21:3950 (1982)
18. J.V. Staros and B.P. Kakkad, Crosslinking and chymotryptic digestion of the extracytoplasmic domain of the anion exchange channel in intact human erythrocytes, J. Membrane Biol. 74:247 (1983)
19. T. Suzuki and G.L. Dale, Biotinylated erythrocytes: *In vivo* survival and *in vitro* recovery, Blood. 70:791 (1987)
20. J. Vaysse ; L. Gattegno; D. Bladier and D. Aminoff, Adhesion and electrophagocytosis of human senescent erythrocytes by autologous monocytes and their inhibition by beta-galactosyl derivatives, Proc. Natl. Acad. Sci. USA 83:1339 (1986)
21. E.Zocchi, M. Tonetti, C. Polvani, L. Guida, U. Benatti and A. DeFlora, Encapsulation of doxorubicin in liver-targeted erythrocytes increases the therapeutic index of the drug in a murine metastatic model, Proc. Natl. Acad. Sci. USA, 86:2040 (1989)
22. L. Zolla, G. Lupidi, M. Marcheggiani, G. Falcioni and M. Brunori, Encapsulation of proteins into human erythrocytes: a kinetic investigation, Biochim. Biophys. Acta 1024:5 (1990)

16

RAT CARRIER ERYTHROCYTES CIRCULATE AND ARRIVE TO ORGANS

F. J. Alvarez, J. A. Jordán, J. C. Murciano, J. Luque, A. Herráez, J. C. Díez, and M. C. Tejedor

Department of Biochemistry and Molecular Biology
University of Alcalá
28871 Alcalá de Henares
Spain

1. INTRODUCTION

Different delivery systems are currently used in therapy. They have the advantage of protecting the active substance from rapid clearance and avoiding toxic side effects. Among the many carrier systems proposed[12], RBCs have many desirable properties: they are naturally biodegradable and may stay in circulation over prolonged periods of time[11,25]; RBCs are easily obtainable and large amounts of material can be entrapped in a small volume of cells by hypotonic dialysis; autologous cells elicit little or no immune response[7,16,20].

Most data support the conclusion that the lysed and resealed RBC may be of large value for carrying drugs in various treatments in different mammalian species[4,8–11,19,22,24] and they have near normal in vivo survival. The disadvantage of the majority of the other encapsulation methods is that the cells loose their viability when returned to the circulation[5].

Rat erythrocytes have not often been used as carriers for therapeutic agents, probably due to unfavourable hemoglobin solubility and membrane properties[15]. Anyhow, we have previously demonstrated that rat RBCs can bind and/or encapsulate substances of different nature and molecular size and we have established both the conditions to prepare and the features of rat carrier erythrocytes[2,3,18,21].

Both radioactive and fluorescent labelling can be usefully applied to detect marker compounds. Radioactive labelling can reveal the presence of the selected substance in RBCs after encapsulation. In our work, Carbonic Anhydrase (CA) was selected for encapsulation because it is a protein available as M_r marker, easy to label with ^{125}I and supposed stable in the intracellular medium. Fluorescently labelled Dextran (FITC-Dx) can be used as a molecular marker for measuring substance uptake since it can not passively enter

Erythrocytes as Drug Carriers in Medicine, edited by Sprandel and Way
Plenum Press, New York, 1997

cells[14] and can help to analyze the biochemical and functional features of subpopulations of loaded RBCs.

Both in human and animals, IP injection of carrier erythrocytes has proved a viable and somewhat advantageous alternative to IV injections[8–10]. We chose to adopt IP administration, since it allows to comparatively study chemically[13] modified loaded rat RBCs.

The present paper intends to review the feasibility of using rat RBCs for encapsulation and delivery of active substances, given the convenience of rat as experimental model in biological assays. Keeping in mind that the most important criterion for RBC viability is survival in circulation, and given the limited number of available "in vivo" studies of carrier rat erythrocytes, the loaded rat RBCs features are examined, as well as their "in vivo" circulation, diffusion of encapsulated ^{125}I-CA, and distribution of both among the different organs that play a role in removal of RBCs.

2. MATERIAL AND METHODS

2.1. Chemicals and Radioisotopes

Carbonic anhydrase (M_r 29000) and FITC-dextran (M_r 19600) were obtained from Sigma Chemical Co. (St. Louis, MO, USA). Na^{125}I (100 mCi/ml) was purchased from NEN Division of Du Pont (Brussels, Belgium). Carbonic anhydrase was iodinated in our laboratory using chloramine-T immobilized on polystyrene beads (Iodo-Beads, Pierce Chemical Co., Rockford, IL, USA). Antibiotic-antimycotic mixture to add to CPDA solution was from Gibco Laboratories (Grand Island, NY, USA). ATP and Glutathione were from Boehringer Mannheim (Germany). Ficoll-Paque was purchased from Pharmacia (Uppsala, Sweden). The dialysis bag was from Medicell (London, UK). Other chemicals used were reagent grade and were purchased from Merck (Darmstadt, Germany).

2.2. Buffers and Solutions

Isotonic (300 mOsm/kg) and hypotonic (80 mOsm/kg) PBS and PBSH solutions, PIGPA and all solutions of ^{125}I-carbonic anhydrase and FITC-dextran were prepared according to previously established conditions[1–3]. CPDA solution was 2.2 mM citric acid, 13.5 mM sodium citrate, 0.2 mM Na_2HPO_4, 2.3 mM dextrose, 0.3 mM adenine, 130 mM NaCl and 1 % antimicrobial mixture.

2.3. Preparation of RBCs

Rat blood (Wistar, 200 g) was collected into heparinized tubes. Blood was centrifuged at 900 g for 5 min and the plasma, white cells and platelets were discarded. RBCs were washed three times in isotonic PBS (pH=8.0). In the last wash each fraction was centrifuged at 2500 g, 5 min to obtain packed RBCs (80% haematocrit).

2.4. Dialysis Loading Procedure

Packed erythrocytes were subjected to the loading procedure according to previously established conditions[2,21]. The marker is added to RBC suspension to final concentration of 34.5 μM ^{125}I-CA (18.82 ± 1.55 · 10^8 cpm/μmol) or 400 μM FITC-Dx. The mixture is dialysed at 4°C for 1 h against hypotonic PBSH (80 mOsm/kg) supplemented with 2 mM ATP and 3 mM GSH. The cells are then annealed (37°C for 10 min) and resealed by 0.5 vol of hypertonic PIGPA solution (37°C for 30 min) and washed three times in cold isotonic PBSH (160 g, 5 min). Aliquots were taken for measurement of gamma-radioactivity or fluorescence. The encapsulation of fluorescent marker (FITC-Dx) was measured by flow cytometry and that of radioactive marker (^{125}I-CA) was determined in a gamma-radiocounter. Control cells, equally processed but in isotonic medium, provided a measurement of non-specific binding of CA and FITC-Dx to RBCs. To study RBC survival and viability after the encapsulation process, the erythrocytes were counted and sized in an haematological analyzer.

2.5. Fluorescence Microscopy

Native, control and loaded cells were examined in an optical fluorescence microscope (Olimpus B071) as fresh preparations without fixation or staining to observe morphological and fluorescence changes due to the method used for loading cells with substances.

2.6. Fractionation of Loaded Rat RBCs Population

2.6.1. Centrifugation on Ficoll-Paque. Control and loaded erythrocytes were fractionated on Ficoll-Paque in order to obtain a more homogeneous population of loaded RBCs. Three volumes of Ficoll-Paque were added to a centrifuge tube and carefully overlaid with four volumes of erythrocyte suspension without mixing them. The system was centrifuged at 400 g for 30 min at 18–20°C and after that, the pellet and supernatant subpopulations were taken and washed three times at 200 g, for 5 min. Both populations were analyzed for cellular parameters and the degree of encapsulation measured by fluorescence microscopy and flow cytometry, or by radioactive counting.

2.6.2. Two-Phase System Partition. 5μl of packed ^{125}I-CA loaded RBCs were added to a PEG/Dx two-phase system[18]. The partition ratio, defined as the amount of cells in the top phase, as a percentage of the total number of cells added, was calculated.

2.7. "*In Vivo*" Assays

2.7.1. ^{51}Cr Labelling. After the resealing step in the loading cell procedure, ^{125}I-CA loaded erythrocytes were incubated with [^{51}Cr]-sodium chromate to radiolabel the haemoglobin as described by Morrison et al.[17]. Loosely packed loaded RBCs were mixed with 50 μl of ^{51}Cr solution (100 μCi/μl) for 30 min at 37°C. Thereafter, cells were washed three to four times in isotonic PBSH to remove unbound ^{51}Cr and used for "in vivo" or "in vitro" experiments. Native RBCs were labelled similarly for control. A 500 μl aliquot of loaded (^{125}I-CA, 2.54 ± 0.09·10^6 cpm) and ^{51}Cr-labelled (2.65 ± 0.16·10^6 cpm) RBC suspension in saline (5 · 10^9 RBCs / ml, 30 % haematocrit) was injected into the intraperitoneal cavity of male Wistar rats (10 weeks old, 250–300 g).

2.7.2. Survival and Organ Uptake of Carrier Rat RBCs. Rats were injected with ^{51}Cr-labelled, either native or loaded, cells. To study the circulation of carrier RBCs, samples of blood (400 µl) were taken from the tail vein of injected animals at designated time points (4–8 rats at each time). Whole blood, cell pellet and plasma were assayed for radioactivity. Cellular recovery (^{51}Cr) and CA (^{125}I) present in circulation were expressed as percent of the amount of radioactivity injected, assuming total blood volume as 6% of body weight. As a control, free ^{125}I-CA was administered by the same route to separate animals.

To study the organ distribution of carrier cells, two rats were killed at each time point by cervical dislocation. The organs were excised, immediately blotted dry and stored at -70°C. Tissues were minced and the total ^{51}Cr and ^{125}I radioactivity in each tissue was determined with different gates in a gamma counter. Results were expressed as percentage of the total injected radioactivity. All experiments were run in triplicate.

3. RESULTS AND DISCUSSION

3.1. Loaded Rat RBCs

The hypotonic encapsulation of several marker substances into rat RBCs has shown that a lower amount of substance is incorporated, as compared to human or other species RBCs[21]. However, since there is a lower cell recovery in rat caused by the encapsulation process, the amount of substance that is encapsulated per cell is similar in rat than in other species[3,21]. Cellular integrity of loaded rat RBCs was revealed through microscope observations after the use of fluorescently labelled marker (FITC-dextran) for the encapsulation (Fig. 1).

These two facts (amount encapsulated and cellular integrity) make possible to think of rat loaded RBCs as feasible drug carriers, according to yields expressed in Table 1.

Other cellular properties of hypotonically loaded rat RBCs have been reported previously[2,3]. In summary, they show increased cell volume (MCV) and higher size dispersion (RDW); this size heterogeneity is also appreciated by flow cytometry analysis[2].

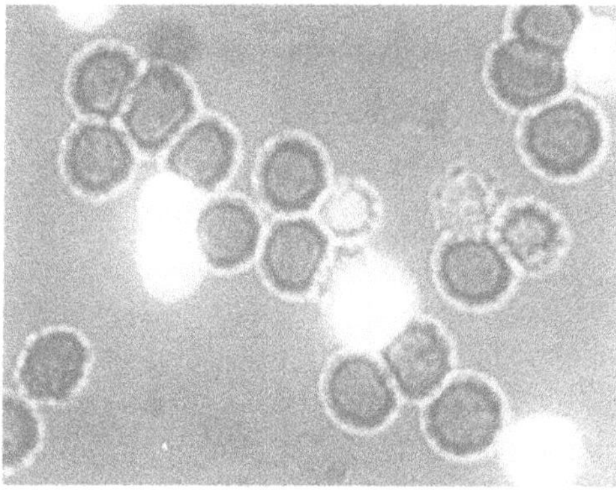

(A) Normal and fluorescence lamps

(B) Fluorescence lamp

Figure 1. Microscopic observation of rat RBCs loaded with FITC-dextran. Left panel shows the cells illuminated with both normal light and fluorescence source (A) and the right panel shows the RBCs illuminated only with fluorescence source (B).

Table 1. Total amount and recovery of cells and radioactive markers all along the encapsulation and labelling processes. The rightmost column shows the overall recovery of cells, iodine and chromium from the starting native RBCs to the final sample injected (i.e. loaded and labelled RBCs)

	Native RBCs	Loaded RBCs	Labelled RBCs	Injected sample
RBCs (10^9/ml)	11.6 ± 0.3	5.7 ± 0.4	4.2 ± 0.3	
Recovery (%)	100	49.3 ± 3.7 100	71.0 ± 4.4	35.3
^{125}I-CA (10^6 cpm/ml)	19.8 ± 0.5	4.8 ± 0.3	3.84 ± 0.34	
Recovery *(%)*	100	23.7 ± 1.4 100	81.3 ± 3.7	19.3
^{51}Cr-RBCs (10^6 cpm/ml)		5.6 ± 0.3	3.56 ± 0.15	
Recovery (%)		100	63.1 ± 3.5	63.12
^{125}I (cpm/10^3 cells)	1.71	0.84	0.91	0.91
^{51}Cr (cpm/10^3 cells)		0.98	0.84	0.84

Heterogeneity is also apparent in terms of encapsulated substance. This cannot be discerned by radioactivity, but is easily appreciated using the fluorescent marker. Two loaded cell populations are evident (Fig. 1), one with high fluorescence content and another with a background staining; the same is shown by flow cytometry[2]. Consistent results are obtained by two-phase system partitioning, which partially discriminates two subpopulations on the basis of their surface properties[18]. On the other hand, density fractionation on Ficoll (Table 2) also produces a major pellet subpopulation (91 % of cells) with the lowest level of encapsulated substance (0.09 cpm/10^3 cells) and a supernatant subpopulation comprising only 8.6 % of loaded cells but with a higher concentration of encapsulated ^{125}I-CA (2.10 cpm/10^3 cells). In any case, the total isolation of two homogeneous populations is not achieved.

3.2. Circulation of Carrier Rat RBCs and Diffusion of CA

"In vivo" behaviour of ^{51}Cr-labelled loaded RBCs is evaluated in comparison to ^{51}Cr-native RBCs (Fig. 2, top panel). Loaded RBCs reach the maximum level in circulation, 50 % versus 85 % for native cells, 24 h after intraperitoneal injection. This important difference in incorporation must be due to modifications introduced by the encapsulation process, corroborating the above-mentioned heterogeneity, that must be affecting the behaviour of loaded RBCs upon crossing the peritoneal barrier.

Table 2. Fractionation by sedimentation on Ficoll-Paque of loaded rat RBCs population. Fractions P and S are, respectively, those which sediment and supernate on Ficoll

Sample	Encapsulated ^{125}I-CA cpm (%)	Cell number (%)	^{125}I-CA concentration (cpm / 10^3 cells) [a]	MCV (fl)	RDW (%)
Loaded	100	100	0.21 ± 0.02	64.6 ± 0.5	22.6 ± 1.2
Fraction "P"	43.3 ± 3.5	91.3 ± 4.3	0.09 ± 0.02	64.6 ± 1.8	22.4 ± 0.6
Fraction "S"	56.7 ± 3.5	8.6 ± 4.3	2.10 ± 0.62	65.7 ± 1.7	35.3 ± 2.5

(a)These experiments were done with a lower specific activity of ^{125}I-CA (18.8 · 10^7 cpm/µmol).

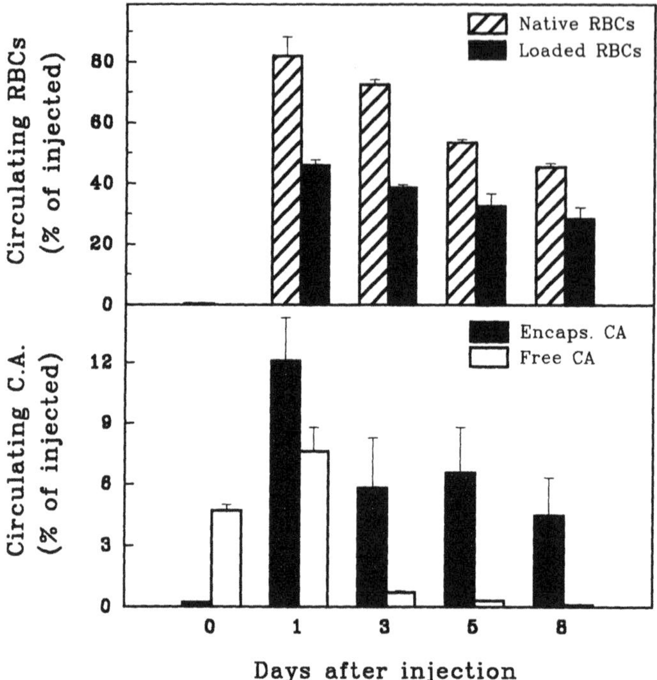

Figure 2. Circulation and disappearance of rat ^{51}Cr-RBCs loaded with ^{125}I-CA. Levels in whole blood of rat are shown. Top panel: presence of ^{51}Cr radioactivity associated to both types of cells, native and loaded. Bottom panel: levels of 125I-CA, administered in free form or in encapsulated form.

Approximately 25 % of the injected loaded RBCs remain in circulation 8–10 days post-injection, indicating an advantageous half-life for carrier rat RBCs. These levels of circulation are comparable to those described for other species[6,8,23].

The encapsulated ^{125}I-CA reaches a reasonable level in circulation (Fig. 2, bottom panel), maintaining significant levels up to 10 days post-injection. In contrast, and as expected[25], CA injected in free form is rapidly incorporated to circulation, metabolized and excreted; only an 8 % is present in blood at 24 h and the level is negligible after 3 days. This demonstrates the stabilization of CA by encapsulation. The maintenance of steady amounts of encapsulated CA in blood indicates that rat RBCs are competent as slow and continuous release agents for exogenous substances in circulation.

3.3. Organ Uptake of Carriers and Delivery of Encapsulated CA

Liver is the organ with higher elimination capacity for both native and loaded cells (Fig. 3, top panel), showing its greatest activity at 24 hours postinjection. The extent of removal is increased for loaded with respect to native cells, mainly in spleen which shows a 5-fold increase in its activity near the 5th day post-injection; similar behaviour has been observed in mice[9]. The uptake capacity of other tissues, such as lungs and kidneys, is also studied, showing little activity both for native and loaded RBCs. The low removal of loaded rat RBCs by tissues agrees with limited "in vitro" recognition of these cells by

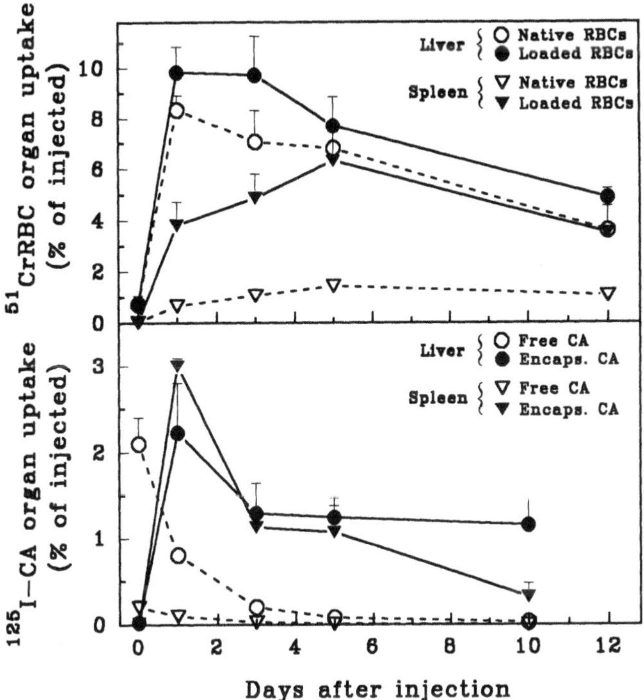

Figure 3. Organ uptake of rat ^{51}Cr-RBCs loaded with ^{125}I-CA. Top panel: increased organ uptake of loaded RBCs with respect to native cells. Bottom panel: comparative arrival to organs of ^{125}I-CA either administered in free form or encapsulated into RBCs.

peritoneal macrophages (preliminary results, Alvarez et al., 24th FEBS Meeting, Barcelona, July 1996).

It is also in the first 24 hours when the highest concentration of ^{125}I-CA is present in all organs studied (Fig. 3, bottom panel), when CA is administered in encapsulated form. In accordance with detectable levels of encapsulated CA found in circulation up to 10 days postinjection, its arrival to liver and spleen is observed until this time. Conversely, CA administered in free form is only present in liver, and only at short times.

An indication of the fate of effectively loaded RBCs is provided by the ratio between ^{125}I (CA) and ^{51}Cr (cells). The highest ratio is showed at 24 h for all organs, indicating a faster removal of the RBCs that have encapsulated more CA. Details about these data have been more extensively discussed[1].

In summary, rat RBCs can be loaded with substances by hypotonic dialysis and isotonic resealing. When these carriers are administered by IP injection they reach an incorporation rate and half-life in circulation that can justify their use as a potential sustained delivery system. They have a capacity for long-term dissemination of drug into the organism with specially increased delivery to spleen. This makes viable the use of rat as an experimental model for biochemical and pharmacological studies in relation to this therapeutic carrier system.

4. ACKNOWLEDGMENTS

This work was supported by grants from the D.G.I.C. y T. (PB 94/0367), U.A.H. (Grant 024/95) and C.I.C.y T. (FAR 90/102). F.J. Alvarez and J.A. Jordán were supported by fellowships from Comunidad Autónoma de Madrid and Universidad de Alcalá de Henares.

5. REFERENCES

1. F.J. Alvarez, A. Herráez, J.C. Murciano, J.A. Jordán, J.C. Díez, and M.C. Tejedor, In vivo survival and organ uptake of loaded carrier rat erythrocytes. J. Biochem. 120:286 (1996).
2. F.J. Alvarez, A. Herráez, and M.C. Tejedor, Fluorescence analysis of carrier rat and human erythrocytes loaded with FITC-dextran. Cytometry 24:181 (1996).
3. F.J. Alvarez, A. Herráez, M.C. Tejedor, and J.C. Díez, Behaviour of isolated rat and human red blood cells upon hypotonic-dialysis encapsulation of carbonic anhydrase and dextran. Biotechnol. Appl. Biochem. 23:173 (1996).
4. U. Benatti, E. Zocchi, M. Tonetti, L. Guida, C. Polvani, and A. De Flora, Enhanced antitumor activity of adriamycin by encapsulation in mouse erythrocytes targeted to liver and lungs. Pharmacol. Res. 21:27 (1989).
5. L. Chiarantini, A. Antonelli, G. Serafini, A. Fraternale, and M. Magnani, In vivo survival and in vitro phagocytosis of engineered erythrocytes. Adv. Biosci. 92:83 (1994).
6. L. Chiarantini, J. Johnson, and J.R. DeLoach, Optimized recirculation survival of mouse carrier erythrocytes. Blood Cells 17:607 (1991).
7. A. De Flora, E. Zocchi, L. Guida, C. Polvani, and U. Benatti, Conversion of encapsulated 5-fluoro-2'-deoxyuridine 5'-monophosphate to the antineoplastic drug 5-fluoro-2'-deoxyuridine in human erythrocytes. Proc. Nat. Acad. Sci. USA 85:3145 (1988).
8. J.R. DeLoach, K. Andrews, W. Satterfield, and M. Keeling, Intraperitoneal administration of carrier erythocytes in dogs: an improved method for delivery of L-asparaginase. Biotechnol. Appl. Biochem. 12:331 (1990).
9. J.R. DeLoach, K. Andrews, and C.L. Sheffield, Encapsulation of interleukin-2 in murine erythrocytes and subsequent deposition in mice receiving a subcutaneous injection. Biotechnol. Appl. Biochem. 10:183 (1988).
10. J.R. DeLoach and R.E. Droleskey, Survival of murine carrier erythrocytes injected via peritoneum. Comp. Biochem. Physiol. A 84:447 (1986).
11. J.R. DeLoach and R.E. Droleskey, Preparation of ovine carrier erythrocytes: their action and survival. Comp. Biochem. Physiol. A 84:441 (1986).
12. P.K. Gupta, Drug targeting in cancer chemotherapy: a clinical perspective. J. Pharm. Sci. 79:949 (1990).
13. J.A. Jordán, R.B. Moyes, R. Droleskey, J.C. Díez, J. Luque, and J.R. DeLoach, In vitro and in vivo evaluation of BS^3 and DTSSP crosslinked erythrocytes. Adv. Biosci. 92:17 (1994).
14. G. Lee, T.M. Delohery, Z. Ronai, P.W. Brandt-Rauf, M.R. Pincus, R.B. Murphy, and I.B. Weinstein, A comparison of techniques for introducing macromolecules into living cells. Cytometry 14:265 (1993).
15. J. Luque, M.I. Garín, S. Sanz, P. Ropero, and M. Pinilla, Properties of hypotonized, crosslinked and crosslinked-permeabilized rat erythrocytes as potential carrier systems. Adv. Exp. Med. Biol. 326:81 (1992).
16. M. Magnani, G. Serafini, and V. Stocchi, Hexokinase type I multiplicity in human erythrocytes. Biochem. J. 254:617 (1988).
17. M. Morrison, A.W. Michaels, D.R. Phillips, and S. Choi, Life span of erythrocyte membrane protein. Nature 248:763 (1974).
18. M.T. Pérez, F.J. Alvarez, A.I. García-Pérez, L. Lucas, M.C. Tejedor, and P. Sancho, Heterogeneity of hypotonically loaded rat erythrocyte populations as detected by counter-current distribution in aqueus polymer two-phase systems. J. Chromatogr. B 677:45 (1996).
19. E. Pitt, C.M. Johnson, D.A. Lewis, D.A. Jenner, and R.E. Offord, Encapsulation of drugs in intact erythrocytes and intravenous delivery system. Biochem. Pharmacol. 32:3359 (1983).
20. L. Rossi, M. Bianchi, A. Fraternale, and M. Magnani, Normalization of hyperglycemia in diabetic mice by enzyme-loaded erythrocytes. Adv. Exp. Med. Biol. 326:183 (1992).

21. M.C. Tejedor, C.E. Alvarez, F.J. Alvarez, A. Herráez, and J. Luque, Comparative encapsulation at different hypotonic pressures in human and rat erythrocytes. Adv. Biosci. 92:73 (1994).
22. M. Tonetti, C. Polvani, E. Zocchi, L. Guida, U. Benatti, P. Biassoni, F. Romei, A. Guglielmi, C. Aschele, A. Sobrero, and A. De Flora, Liver targeting of autologous erythrocytes loaded with doxorubicin. Eur. J. Cancer 27:947 (1991).
23. E. Zocchi, L. Guida, U. Benatti, M. Canepa, L. Borgiani, T. Zanin, and A. De Flora, Hepatic or splenic targeting of carrier erythrocytes: a murine model. Biotechnol. Appl. Biochem. 9:423 (1987).
24. E. Zocchi, M. Tonetti, C. Polvani, L. Guida, U. Benatti, and A. De Flora, In vivo liver and lung targeting of adriamycin encapsulated in glutaraldehyde-treated murine erythrocytes. Biotechnol. Appl. Biochem. 10:555 (1988).
25. L. Zolla, G. Lupidi, M. Marcheggiani, G. Falcioni, and M. Brunori, Encapsulation of proteins into human erythrocytes: a kinetic investigation. Biochim. Biophys. Acta 1024:5 (1990).

17

ENCAPSULATION OF ALCOHOL DEHYDROGENASE AND ACETALDEHYDE DEHYDROGENASE INTO HUMAN ERYTHROCYTES BY AN ELECTROPORATION PROCEDURE

Carmen Lizano, Silvia Sanz, Pilar Sancho, José Luque, and Montserrat Pinilla

Dpto. Bioquímica y Biología Molecular
Campus Universitario, Univ. de Alcalá
28871 Alcalá de Henares
Madrid, Spain

1. SUMMARY

The optimal conditions for electroporation/resealing loading of alcohol dehydrogenase (ADH) and acetaldehyde dehydrogenase (ALDH) into human erythrocytes were first established (37ºC, 300V, 1ms pulse time, 8 pulses every 15min, and 1h resealing). At a fixed enzyme level (100U ADH or 3U ALDH per mL erythrocyte suspension), the encapsulation yield was 26.2% for ADH and 38.3% for ALDH. Carrier cell recoveries were 82–85%. Cell volumes increase while hemoglobin content decrease as a consequence of the electroporation/resealing process (i.e. a decreased cell hemoglobin concentration). Although a lower hypotonic resistance of loaded erythrocytes (all along the osmotic fragility curves) was observed, the non-alteration of the oxygen transport capability (as given by the oxygen equilibrium curves) suggest the electroporation/resealing process as a convenient alternative to the hypotonic-dialysis method for the preparation of ADH- and ALDH-erythrocytes.

2. INTRODUCTION

Different techniques have been used to introduce exogenous substances into red blood cells (RBCs). The potential use of carrier human RBCs for the administration of a variety of substances of therapeutic or biotechnological interest has been largely investigated. Erythrocyte-encapsulated enzymes have been proposed in enzyme-replacement therapy for inborn metabolic errors, as well as bio-reactors for the enzymic degradation of

Erythrocytes as Drug Carriers in Medicine, edited by Sprandel and Way
Plenum Press, New York, 1997

abnormally elevated plasma metabolites[2,3,4,14,17,22]. The electroporation procedure has been employed for the encapsulation of foreign molecules in different cell types, including RBCs. The method is based on the decrease of cell membrane barrier function by exposing cells to a strong electric field pulse (electropermeabilization). The increase in the permeability of the RBC membrane is consistent with the pore formation. The membrane rupture depends on the voltage applied and on the duration of the pulse. If the electric field strength and the exposure time do not exceed critical values, the breakdown is completely reversible[10,11,12,15,20,21].

Loading of RBCs with the enzymes mainly responsible of ethanol degradation in liver (alcohol dehydrogenase, ADH (EC.1.1.1.1), which catalyzes the oxidation of ethanol with reduction of NAD^+, and acetaldehyde dehydrogenase, ALDH (EC.1.2.1.5) which further metabolyzes acetaldehyde), have been achieved using the hypotonic dialysis/isotonic resealing procedure. From these studies, both ADH-RBCs[18,19] and ALDH-RBCs[13,14,16] can be proposed as circulating bio-reactors for the removal of high levels of blood ethanol and acetaldehyde, respectively.

As a further step to this aim, the incorporation of both enzymes into human RBCs using an electroporation procedure, and some basic properties of the carrier RBCs (erythrocyte indexes, hypoosmotic resistance and hemoglobin oxygenation capability) have been examined. This work open the possibility of using electroporated/resealed ADH- and ALDH-RBCs to metabolize the excess of alcohol in blood. The administration of these carrier RBCs may contribute to avoid the damage caused to the liver by ethanol intake.

3. MATERIALS AND METHODS

3.1. Chemicals

Crystallized-lyophilized baker yeast ADH and ALDH were from Sigma-Aldrich Quimica, Spain. Chemicals were of the highest purity available.

3.2. RBC Suspensions

Human blood was drawn from healthy donors by venipuncture into heparinized tubes (10U/mL). The blood was centrifuged (1000xg, 10min, 4ºC) and the plasma and buffy coat removed. RBCs were washed three times in isotonic Hanks-PBS (136.8mmol/L NaCl, 5.3mmol/L KCl, 0.43mmol/L Na_2HPO_4, 0.43mmol/L KH_2PO_4, 1.5mmol/L $MgCl_2$, 0.83mmol/L $MgSO_4$ and 6mmol/L glucose, pH 7.4). In the last wash the cell suspension was centrifuged to obtain packed RBCs (>70% hematocrit).

Different RBC suspensions were prepared: native RBCs in the absence (Control) and in the presence of enzymes (Non-specific binding), and electroporated/resealed RBCs in the absence (Unloaded) and in the presence of enzymes (Loaded).

3.3. Electroporation of ADH and ALDH

Packed RBCs were precisely adjusted to 50% hematocrit with Hanks-PBS, and ADH or ALDH were added to obtain a final activity of 100U/mL or 3U/mL RBCs, respectively. For encapsulation, 0.4mL of these mixtures where place in the cuvette (0.2cm gap). Electroporation was carried out using a BTX Electrosquareporator T820 apparatus (BTX

INC., San Diego, CA, USA). The voltage and duration of the pulse were automatically selected. Experimental conditions are given in Results and Discussion section.

3.4. Erythrocytes Indexes

RBC counts (cells/L), hematocrit (Hct), mean cell volume (MCV), mean cell hemoglobin (MCH) and mean cell hemoglobin concentration (MCHC) were measured with an Hematology Analyzer System 9000 (Serono-Baker Diagnostic, Allentown, PA, USA). Total hemoglobin, oxyhemoblobin (O_2Hb), carboxyhemoglobin (COHb) and methemoglobin (MetHb) were measured with a Co-oximeter IL 482 (Instrumentation Laboratory, Lexington, MA, USA).

3.5. Enzyme Activities

ADH activity was assayed according to Kennedy & Tipton[9]. ALDH activity was assayed according to Bostian & Betts[1] as suggested to us by Sigma Chemical Co., St Louis, MO, USA. Encapsulation (entrapment) is defined by the amount of enzymes that enter into RBCs as a result of the porous stage created during the electroporation process and remain within the cells after the resealing stage. The yield of encapsulation (percentage) is given by the enzyme activity within resealed cells, referred to the initial enzyme activity added to the RBC suspension before electroporation (100%).

3.6. Osmotic-Fragility Curves (OFC) of RBC Suspensions

OFCs were obtained as previously described[19]. The hemolysis of RBCs (50% Hct) in NaCl solutions (up to 300mOsm/Kg, 4ºC, 30min) is given by absorbance values (hemoglobin, 540nm) in the supernatants after centrifugation (1000xg, 5min). The percentage of hemolysis is referred to the absorbance value in water (total hemolysis). Osmolarity was determined by freezing point depression using a Micro-Osmometer (3MO) apparatus (Advanced Instruments, Needham Heights., MA, USA). H_{50} values show the degree of osmolarity required for 50% hemolysis.

3.7. Oxyhemoglobin Dissociation Curves

The oxygen equilibrium curves for the different cell suspensions were automatically recorded in a TCS Hemox Analyzer (TCS Medical Products Co., Southampton, PA, USA) in Hanks-PBS solution, pH 7.4 at 37ºC. P_{50} values show the O_2 partial pressure required for 50% saturation of hemoglobin.

4. RESULTS AND DISCUSSION

4.1. Loading of Erythrocytes with ADH and ALDH

4.1.1. Preliminary Kinetic Study of ALDH. The aim of this work was to encapsulate liver alcohol-metabolic enzymes. However, hepatic ADH or ALDH are not readily available. Enzyme preparations from a different origin (baker yeast), with similar kinetic characteristics to those of hepatic origin, have been here used. The commercial ADH (high-Km 1.3 10^{-2}M) can be used as representative of the liver enzyme. However, different kinetic forms of ALDH are found. The high-Km form of ALDH detected in human RBCs is not adequate to remove acetaldehyde levels in blood after alcohol intake. Therefore, a low-Km form of yeast ALDH (similar to that of mitochondrial hepatic origin)[8,25,26] can be used. In order to confirm that the kinetic parameters of this commercial ALDH is appropriate, a kinetic study was previously carried out. As shown in Fig 1, the Km value thus obtained (132μM) is rather similar to that of ALDH from mitochondrial hepatocites (50μM)[26]. In view of its high substrate affinity for acetaldehyde, this enzyme preparation may be then adequate to be used to remove acetaldehyde after encapsulation.

4.1.2. Electroporation Procedure. In order to optimize the method for the encapsulation of ADH (100U/mL) and ALDH (3U/mL) into human RBCs, studies were carried out in which the experimental parameters involved in electroporation were systematically varied. These were based on the information available for encapsulation of different substances in RBCs[5,6,10,11,12,15,20,21,23,24]. Variations in the voltage applied (200–2200V), pulse length (0.4–1ms), number of pulses (1–8) and resealing conditions (20h at 4ºC and 1h at 37ºC) were studied (results not shown). As a consequence of this study, the parameters selected for electroporation were: 300V, 1ms and 8 pulses every 15min, at 37ºC, followed by resealing (1h incubation at 37ºC). The cells were finally washed three times with isotonic Hanks-PBS (1000xg, 10min, 4ºC).

4.1.3. Encapsulation Parameters and Erythrocyte Indexes for ADH- and ALDH-RBCs (Table I). First, as a control of the electroporation/resealing process, native RBCs were studied (column 1). A "non-specific binding" control was also carried out (column 2), to establish the potential binding of externally added enzymes to the cell surface (and/or their free entrance into the cell). As expected, non detectable specific enzymes binding were observed. The values for cell recovery and erythrocyte indexes were also not varied in both populations.

Second, the results for loaded RBCs (ADH-RBCs, column 4; or ALDH-RBCs, column 5) are shown in Table I in comparison with those for unloaded electroporated/resealed RBCs in the absence of enzymes (column 3). As can be seen, non-significant variations in cell recoveries were observed for loaded or unloaded RBCs (82.8–85.9%). These values were rather high if compared with cell recoveries for the native, non electroporeated/resealed RBCs (98.1–97.6%). Enzyme-entrapment (encapsulation yield) values observed for ADH (26.2%) and ALDH (38.3%) are significantly higher than those ob-

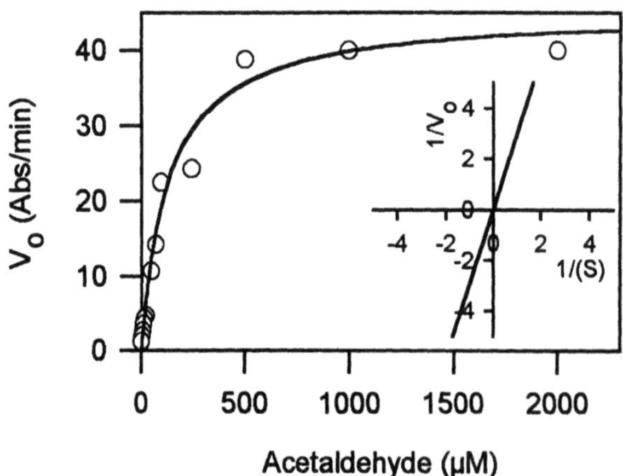

Figure 1. Hyperbolic acetaldehyde saturation curve and double reciproques representation (insert in figure) for the low-Km ALDH from bakers yeast. The calculated Km value is around 132 μM.

tained for human RBCs when using the hypotonic-dialysis/isotonic-resealing procedure (17.2% for ADH[19] and 21% for ALDH[14]).

Third, erythrocyte indexes, which have not been previously studied in electroporated/resealed RBCs, are also shown in Table I. MCV values for unloaded (101.3L), ADH-RBCs (89.7L) and ALDH-RBCs 106.2%) seem to be higher than those observed for native RBCs (85.6–86.1L, in Table I and 88–90L in previous publications[14,19]). Such an increase in cell volume is in contrast with the decrease in cell volume observed after the hypotonic-dialysis/resealing procedure[16,19]. We have no explanation for this data. Also interesting is the apparent decrease in hemoglobin content (MCH) observed in electroporated/resealed RBCs (columns 4–6), in comparison with native control ones (columns 1 and 2). This is due to the loss of hemoglobin through the membrane pores opened during the electroporation process. It should be remind that a non-variation of MCH values is normally observed under the hypotonic/resealing procedure[7,18,19]. As a consequence of the high cell volumes and the lower cell hemoglobin content, the mean cell hemoglobin concentration (MCHC) of electroporated/resealed RBCs is also decreased, in comparison with native RBCs, in Table I.

Finally, the hemoglobin-derivative forms were measured in native-, unloaded-, and ADH- or ALDH-loaded RBCs (results not shown). In general, the high percentages of O_2Hb (95%), the low percentage of COHb (0.5%), and the non-detectable MetHb levels are clearly indicating that the oxygen hemoglobin binding has not been affected by the electroporation/resealing treatment. It means that hemoglobin is completely functional in these carrier RBCs.

4.2. Osmotic Fragility of Human Carrier RBCs

The OFCs are usually studied to establish the hypotonic resistance of carrier RBCs. As shown in Fig 2, the OFCs for native RBCs and electroporated/resealed unloaded- or loaded-RBCs have a different pattern than the dialysed/resealed RBCs[18,19]. The curves for electroporated/resealed RBCs are shifted towards the right (higher H_{50} values) of the curves for native RBCs. This is clearly observed all along the osmotic gradient. It should

Table 1. Encapsulation parameters and erythrocytes indexes for ADH and ALDH carrier human RBCs loaded by electroporation under the following conditions: 300 V, 8 pulses every 15 min at 37ºC, time of pulse 1 ms, resealed cells at 37ºC 1 hr. Other experimental details are given in the text. n=number of experiments (mean±S.E.M.) . Abbreviation: ND, not detectable

			Electroporated/resealed RBCs		
	Native RBCs			Encapsulation	
Parameter	Control	Non-specific binding	Unloaded	ADH	ALDH
n	6	6	4	4	4
Cell Recovery (%)	98.1±0.5	97.6±1.3	83.6±0.8	85.9±0.3	82.8±0.7
Entrapment ADH (%)	—	ND	—	26.2±1.9	—
Entrapment ALDH (%)	—	ND	—	—	38.3±0.8
MCV (fl)	85.6±3.5	86.1±1.8	101.3±2.3	89.7±0.4	106.2±0.9
MCH (pg)	28.9±0.8	30.1±0.9	26.9±1.5	15.9±0.1	22.2±1.5
MCHC (g/dl)	33.8±4.5	33.9±0.7	26.5±2.8	17.8±0.2	20.9±1.3

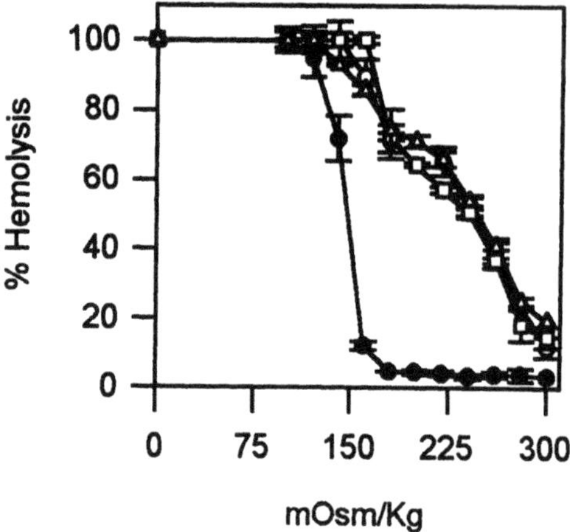

Figure 2. Osmotic-fragility curves (OFC) of human RBC suspensions for: native RBCs (●), and electroporated unloaded (O), ADH-loaded (□) and ALDH-loaded (Δ) RBCs. The H_{50} values are 148mOsm/Kg for native RBCs, and 249, 246 and 247mOsm/Kg for unloaded, ADH-RBCs and ALDH-RBCs mOsm/Kg, respectively.

means that electroporated/resealed RBCs are heterogeneous population as well as more fragile than native RBCs. It should be remind that dialysed/resealed RBCs are also heterogeneous but contain a small fraction of fragile RBCs and a large population of resistant RBCs. The higher fragility of the whole electroporated/resealed RBC population seems to be in agreement with the higher cell volume previously observed (Table I). The differences in hypoosmotic behaviour, which may be a consequence of different encapsulation effects on cell/membrane structure, may be an interesting point for further studies.

4.3. Oxyhemoglobin Dissociation Properties

As shown in Fig. 3, native, unloaded- and ADH- or ALDH-RBCs show similar sigmoidal oxyhemoglobin dissociation curves, with Hill' s coefficient very close to those for native RBCs (**n** around 2). This is indicative of a positive cooperativity in the oxygen binding to hemoglobin. This is not the case in dialyzed/resealed RBCs, in which an increase in oxygen affinity is observed (R. Lopez, unpublished work). Such an important observation is supporting the complete functionality of hemoglobin in our carrier RBCs, as previously suggested in Section 4.1.3.

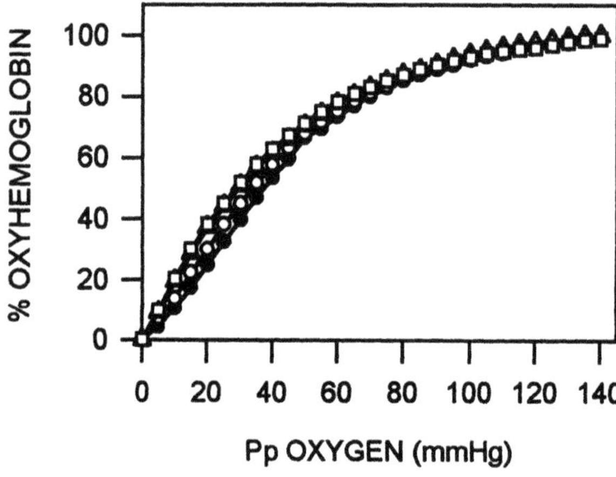

Figure 3. Oxyhemoglobin dissociation curves of human erythrocytes for native RBCs (●), electroporated unloaded (O), ADH-loaded (□) and ALDH-loaded (Δ) RBCs. The P_{50} values are 36mmHg for native RBCs and 34, 31 and 30mmHg for unloaded, ADH loaded and ALDH-loaded RBCs, respectively.

5. REFERENCES

1. Bostian, K.A. and Betts, G.F. (1978) *Biochemical Journal* **173,** 773–786
2. DeLoach, J.R. (1986) Carrier erythrocytes. *Med. Res. Rev.* **6,** 487–504
3. DeLoach, J.R. and Sprandel, U. Eds. (1985) *Red Blood Cells and Carriers for Drugs*. Krager, Basilea
4. DeLoach, J.R. and Way, J.L Eds. (1994) Carrier and Bioreactor red blood cells for drug delivery and targeting. *Adv. Biosci.* **92** Pergamon, Great Britain.
5. Flynn, G., Hackett, T.J. McHale, L. and McHale, A.P. (1994) Encapsulation of the thrombolytic enzyme, brinase, in photosentitized erythrocytes: a novel throbolytic system based on photodynamic activation. *J. of Photochem. and Photobiol. B:Biol.* **26,** 193–196
6. Flynn, G., McHale, L. and McHale, A.P. (1994) Methotrexate-loaded, photosensitized erythrocytes: a photo-activable carrier/delivery system for use in cancer therapy. *Cancer Letters* **82,** 225–229
7. Garin, M., Rossi, L., Luque, J. and Magnani, M. (1995) Lactate catabolism by enzyme-loaded red blood cells. *Biotechnol. Appl. Biochem.* **22,** 295–303
8. Inoue K., Nishimukai, M. and Yamasawa, K. (1979) Purification and partial characterization of the aldehyde dehydrogenase from human RBCs. *Biochim. Biophys. Acta* **569,** 117–123
9. Kennedy, N.P. and Tipton, K.F. (1990) Ethanol metabolism and alcoholic liver disease. *Assay Biochem.* **25,** 137–195
10. Kinosita, K. and Tsong, T.Y. (1977) Formation and resealing of pores of controlled sizes in human erythrocyte membrane. *Nature* **268,** 438–441.
11. Kinosita, K. Tsong, T.Y. and Tsong, Jr. (1977) Voltage-induced pore formation and hemolysis of human erythrocytes. *Biochim. Biophys. Acta.* **471,** 227–242
12. Magal, P.c. and Kaur, A. (1991) Electroporation of red blood cell membrane and its use as a drug carrier system. *Indian J. Biochem & Biophys.* **28,** 219–221
13. Magnani, M., Laguerre, M., Rossi, L., Bianchi, M., Ninfali, P., Magnani, F. and Ropars, C. (1990) In *vivo* accelerated acetaldehyde metabolism using acetaldehyde dehydrogenase-loaded erythrocytes. *Alcohol and Alcoholism.* **25,**627–637
14. Magnani, M. and DeLoach, J.R. Eds. (1992) The Use of Resealed Erythrocytes as Carriers and Bioreactors *Adv. Exp. Med. Biol.* **326,** Plenum Press, New York.
15. Mouneimne, Y., Barhoumi, R., Myers, S., Slogoff, S. and Nicolau, C. (1990) Stable rightward shiths of the oxyhemoglobin dissociation curves induced by encapsulation of inositol hexaphosphate in red blood cells using electroporation. *FEBS LETTERS* **275,** 117–120
16. Ninfali, P., Rossi, L., Baronciani, Tirillini, B., Ropars, C. and Magnani, M. (1992) Acetaldehyde, ethanol and acetate concentration in blood of alcohol-treated mice receiving aldehyde dehydrogenase-loaded erythrocytes. *Alcohol and Alcoholism,* **27,** 19–23.
17. Ropars, C., Chassaigne, M. and Nicolau, C. Eds. (1987) *Red blood cells as a carriers for drug. Pergamon,* Oxford
18. Sanz, S., Lizano, C., Garín, M. and Pinilla, M. (1996) *In vitro* studies on alcohol and glutamate dehydrogenase encapsulated into erythrocytes. This meeting.
19. Sanz, S., Pinilla, M. Garín, M., Tipton, K.F. and Luque, J. (1995) The influence of enzyme concentration on the encapsulation of glutamate dehydrogenase and alcohol dehydrogenase in red blood cells *Biotechnol. Appl. Biochem.* **22,** 223–231
20. Saulis, G., Venslauskas, M.S. and Naktinis, J. (1991) Kinetics of pore resealing in cell membranes after electroporation. *J. Electroanal. Chem.* **321,** 1–13
21. Serpersu, E.H., Kinosita, K.Jr. and Tsong, T.Y. (1985) Reversible and irreversible modification of erythrocyte membrane permeability by electric field. *Biochim. bioph. Acta.* **812,** 779–785
22. Tonetti, M., De Flora, A. (1993) Carrier erythrocytes. Clinical pharmacokinetic considerations. *Clin. Pharmacokinet.* **25(5),** 351–357
23. Wu, Y., Sifri, C.D., Lei, H., Su, X. and Wellems, T.E. (1995), Transfection of *Plasmodium falciparum* within human red blood cells. *Proc. Natl. Acad. Sci.* **92,** 973–977
24. Zimmermann, U., Riemann, R. and Ritwat, G. (1976) Enzyme loading of electrically homogeneous human red blood cell ghosts prepared by dielectric breakdown. *Biochim. Biophyd. Acta.* **436,** 460–474
25. Zorzano, A. and Herrera, E. (1990) Differences in the kinetic properties and sensitivity to inhibitors of human placental, erythrocyte, and major hepatic aldehyde dehydrogenase isoenzymes. *Biochem. Pharmacol.* **39,** 873
26. Zorzano, A. Ruiz del Arbol, L. and Herrera, E. (1989) Effect of liver disorders on ethanol elimination and alcohol and aldehyde dehydrogenase activities in liver and erythrocytes. *Clinical Science* **76,** 51–57

18

PHARMACOKINETICS OF DOXORUBICIN IN PATIENTS WITH LYMPHOPROLIFERATIVE DISORDERS AFTER INFUSION OF DOXORUBICIN-LOADED ERYTHROCYTES

Fazoil I. Ataullakhanov, Valentin G. Isaev, Alina V. Kohno, Elena V. Kulikova, Elena N. Parovichnikova, Valery G. Savchenko, and Victor M. Vitvitsky

Scientific Center for Hematology of RAMS
125167 Moscow, Russia

1. ABSTRACT

Pharmacokinetics of doxorubicin infused as a solution or doxorubicin-loaded erythrocytes was studied in three patients with lymphoproliferative disorders. Homologous or autologous erythrocytes were loaded with doxorubicin aseptically by their incubation at 37°C in the solution of doxorubicin for 1 h. During the i.v. infusion of doxorubicin in solution (25–50 mg per square meter of body surface area), its concentration in blood rose to 3.60–5.90 ug/ml. Doxorubicin declined to about 0.1 ug/ml 20–30 min postinfusion and became zero 12–24 hours later. When these patients received the same doses of doxorubicin loaded into erythrocytes, doxorubicin in blood did not exceed 2.5 ug/ml. Within 10–30 min after the end of the infusion, doxorubicin decreased to about 0.1 ug/ml and remained at this level for 3 days and longer. Administrations of doxorubicin-loaded erythrocytes produced no adverse side effects.

2. INTRODUCTION

Anthracycline antibiotics are potent anticancer agents that are broadly used for treatment of various malignant diseases. However, their high toxicity may cause severe adverse effects[7,14,16,18]. The use of erythrocytes as carriers of anthracycline antibiotics is promising for decreasing antibiotic toxicity and increasing its specific activity. Under certain conditions, intact erythrocytes can bind considerable amounts of anthracycline antibiotics[2,4,5,19,20]. However, this binding is weak and the antibiotics easily leave the erythrocytes[3,8,11,19,21]. It is possible to immobilize anthracycline antibiotics within erythrocytes by glutaraldehyde[3,9,19,21]. The use of

Erythrocytes as Drug Carriers in Medicine, edited by Sprandel and Way
Plenum Press, New York, 1997

doxorubicin-loaded erythrocytes (DLE) increases the lifetime of the antibiotic in the circulation and can provide target delivery of this antibiotic to spleen, liver, and lungs decreasing the antibiotic burden for other organs[10,15,21]. DLE were superior to the standard doxorubicin preparation in suppressing liver metastases in mice[22]. A clinical attempt to treat massive liver metastases with DLE was reported[20]. DLE were also used to treat lymphosarcoma in dogs[15]. However, along with high anticancer activity, DLE displayed pronounced myelotoxicity that caused severe pancytopenia in dogs[15]. In the cited studies, doxorubicin was immobilized in erythrocytes with glutaraldehyde. Glutaraldehyde treatment is likely to modify doxorubicin and this modification is associated with an uncontrollable change in the antibiotic toxicity. However, the efficacy of erythrocytes loaded with anthracycline antibiotics seems to be independent of how tightly antibiotics are bound within cells. Daunorubicin-loaded erythrocytes prepared without glutaraldehyde treatment were shown to display higher anticancer activity[11,12] and lower toxicity[1] than daunorubicin in solution. Therefore, it is a plausible suggestion that erythrocytes loaded with doxorubicin without glutaraldehyde treatment will also be superior to doxorubicin in solution.

This study is the first step of the clinical trial of DLE prepared without glutaraldehyde treatment and is aimed at evaluating their pharmacokinetics and tolerance.

3. MATERIALS AND METHODS

Three patients with lymphoproliferative disorders were studied. All they received chemotherapy according to the protocol involving doxorubicin treatment. Patient characteristics are briefly summarized in Table 1.

We used adriablastin produced by Farmitalia Carlo Erba (Montedison Group, Italy) for infusion as solution (standard form) and for preparation of DLE. To prepare DLE we dissolved the desired amount of adriablastin in physiological saline (70 ml) and introduced it into the blood bag containing packed erythrocytes (200 ml) preheated to 37°C. Erythrocytes were either homologous (for patient A) or autologous (patients B and C). After being thoroughly mixed, cells were incubated at 37°C for 1 h. These temperature and time of incubation provided almost complete binding of the antibiotic[4,20]. At the end of incubation, saline (100 ml) was added into the bag. All the manipulations were performed under sterile conditions. The suspension of DLE was infused to the patient immediately after preparation.

We studied the pharmacokinetics of doxorubicin in each patient on two separate occasions. In the first study, the patient received a single standard dose of doxorubicin in so-

Table 1. Characteristics of patients

Patient	A	B	C
Sex	F	M	M
Age	63	21	16
Diagnosis	Lymph.[a]	Lymphog [b]	Lymphog [b]
Disease stage	IV	IVBb	IVBb
Chemotherapy protocol including doxorubicin	CHOP	ABVD	ABVD
The number of chemotherapy cycles preceding the infusion of DLE	3	3	1
Doxorubicin per infusion (mg/m^2)	50	25	25

[a]Lymph. is the abreviation of Lymphosarcoma
[b]Lymphog. is the abreviation of Lymphogranulomatosis

lution. In the second study, this patient received the same dose of doxorubicin through the infusion of DLE. Patient A was treated with doxorubicin in solution and DLE within the two consecutive cycles of CHOP. Patients B and C received infusions of both types within one cycle of ABVD. Standard doxorubicin in solution and suspension of DLE were infused into the cubital vein for 10 min and 1–3 h, respectively. The first sample of blood for doxorubicin determination was drawn immediately after the end of the infusion. Further blood sampling was performed at various time intervals within 3 days postinfusion. Blood-preserving solution Glugicir, an analog of ACD, was used for anticoagulation. Each blood sample was split into two portions. One portion was immediately frozen. The second portion was centrifuged, and the supernatant plasma was separated from cells and frozen. Frozen samples of blood and plasma were stored at -20°C.

Blood and plasma samples were thawed, and 1.6 M K_2CO_3 (0.1 ml) and chloroform (3 ml) was added to 1 ml of the sample. The mixture was vigorously stirred and centrifuged at 1000 g for 3 min. The chloroform extract of doxorubicin at the bottom of the tube was carefully collected with a glass syringe. Doxorubicin in the chloroform extracts was determined spectrofluorometrically (476-nm excitation and 588-nm emission). Solutions of doxorubicin in chloroform of the known concentrations were used for calibration. The lower detection limit of the method was approximately 10 ng/ml blood or plasma.

4. RESULTS

Despite significant individual differences, the pharmacokinetics of doxorubicin in different patients displayed several general features in common (Fig. 1). Immediately after the end of the infusion of the doxorubicin solution, its concentration in the blood was 3.6–5.9 ug/ml. Doxorubicin sharply declined within 30 min postinfusion by 30-fold or greater and remained at the level of approximately 0.1 ug/ml for several hours. The concentration of doxorubicin fell to zero 12–24 hours postinfusion. When the same doses of doxorubicin were infused loaded in erythrocytes, the pharmacokinetics changed dramatically (Fig. 1). Immediately after the end of the infusion, blood doxorubicin was significantly lower (1.44–2.5 ug/ml) than that after infusion of doxorubicin solution. Within 10–30 min after the end of the infusion of DLE, blood doxorubicin also sharply decreased; however, it remained at the level of 0.1 ug/ml throughout the observation period being nonzero even at 72 h postinfusion. Blood and plasma pharmacokinetics of doxorubicin did not differ.

The different pharmacokinetics of doxorubicin delivered as solution or DLE resulted in the significant differences in the areas under the pharmacokinetic curves (Table 2). In the case of DLE, the 72-h area is several times larger than that observed after the infusion of doxorubicin solution. Patients well tolerated DLE. No immediate or postinfusion adverse reactions were noticed.

5. DISCUSSION

The pharmacokinetic curves for doxorubicin solution observed in this study are similar to those reported by others[6,13,20]. The use of DLE significantly changed the pharmacokinetics of blood doxorubicin. In our opinion, the main difference is a manyfold increase in the circulation time of the antibiotic. Similarly increased circulation times of doxorubicin were observed in dogs that received erythrocytes loaded with doxorubicin and treated with glutaraldehyde[10,15]. In these experiments, blood doxorubicin remained at a level lower than

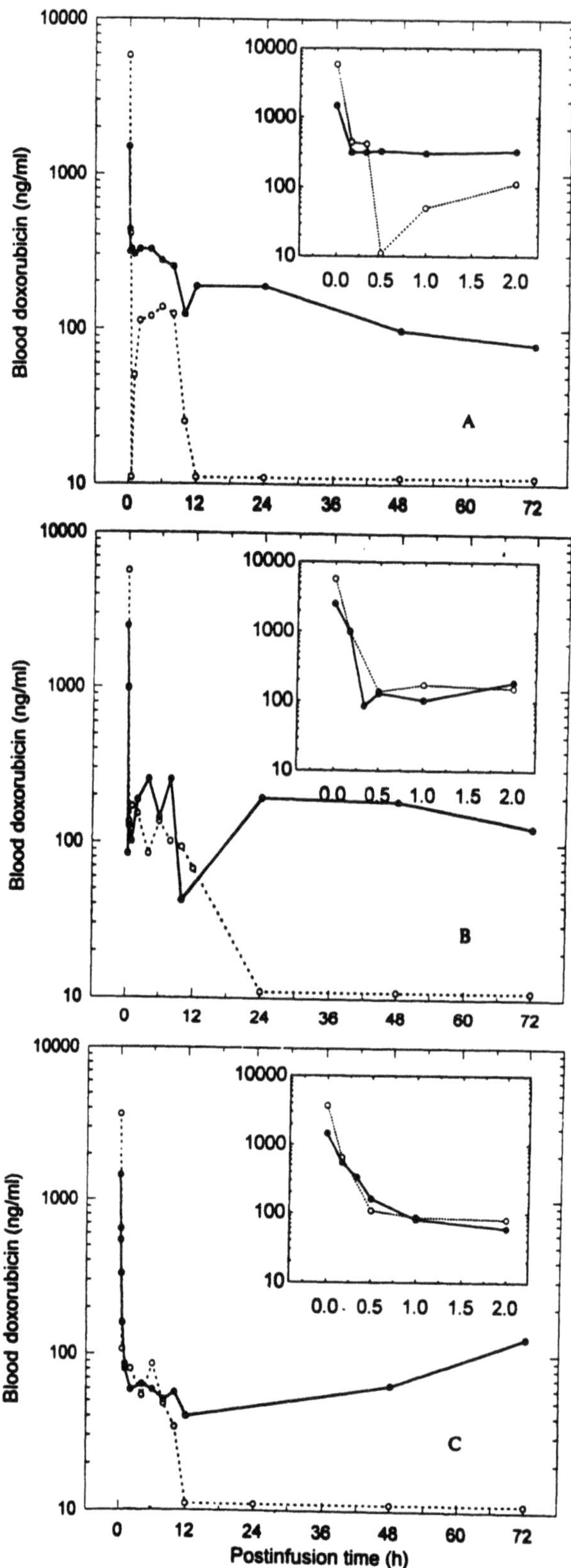

Figure 1. Individual kinetics of blood doxorubicin after infusion of its solution (open circles) or doxorubicin-loaded erythrocytes (dark circles) in (A) patient A, (B) patient B, and (C) patient C. Portions of curves showing the first 2 h postinfusion are in separate frames.

Table 2. The area under the pharmacokinetic curve as a function of time elapsed from the infusion of doxorubicin solution or doxorubicin-loaded erythrocytes (DLE). The areas were calculated from data presented in Fig. 1

	Area under curve (ug h/ml)					
	Patient A		Patient B		Patient C	
Postinfusion time (h:min)	Doxorubicin solution	DLE	Doxorubicin solution	DLE	Doxorubicin solution	DLE
00:00	0.0	0.0	0.0	0.0	0.0	0.0
00:10	0.524	0.150	0.555	0.288	0.357	0.165
00:20	0.595	0.202	-	0.377	-	0.238
00:30	0.628	0.255	0.742	0.395	0.482	0.278
01:00	0.642	0.412	0.818	0.452	0.530	0.338
02:00	0.722	0.678	0.978	0.597	0.613	0.408
04:00	0.953	1.24	1.22	1.04	0.747	0.530
06:00	1.21	1.83	1.44	1.44	0.887	0.653
08:00	1.47	2.37	1.67	1.83	1.02	0.763
10:00	1.62	2.73	1.87	2.13	1.10	0.872
12:00	1.65	3.05	2.03	-	1.14	0.968
24:00	1.65	5.28	2.44	3.79	1.14	-
48:00	1.65	8.70	2.44	8.36	1.14	2.84
72:00	1.65	10.85	2.44	12.12	1.14	5.16

the level that we observed in our patients. It should be noted, however, that we determined doxorubicin from the total fluorescence of samples, and it remained uncertain whether only doxorubicin or doxorubicin and products of its metabolism were present in the samples. Nevertheless, our results suggest that the use of DLE prepared without the tight immobilization of the antibiotic within the cell by glutaraldehyde is highly promising. The technique for preparing such erythrocytes is very simple. Their use allows doxorubicin to circulate significantly longer and thereby may significantly enhance its therapeutic efficacy. In addition, the loaded erythrocytes prepared without glutaraldehyde treatment are better tolerated than those treated with glutaraldehyde. Administration of glutaraldehyde-treated erythrocytes is sometimes associated with adverse side effects[17,20].

6. ACKNOWLEDGMENTS

The authors wish to thank Dr. R.I. Volkova for help in the manuscript preparation.

7. REFERENCES

1. Ataullakhanov, F.I., Batasheva, T.V., Bukhman, V.M., Komarova, S.V., Oreshkina, T.D. and Vitvitsky, V.M. [1994] Treatment of Rausher virus induced murine erythroblastic leukemia with rubomycin loaded erythrocytes, in Carrier and Bioreactor Red Blood Cells for Drug Delivery andTargeting (DeLoach, J.R. and Way, J.L. eds.)., pp. 177–183. Elsevier Science Ltd, Oxford
2. Ataullakhanov, F.I., Batasheva, T.V. and Vitvitsky, V.M. [1994] Influence of temperature, daunorubicin concentration and suspension hematocrit on daunorubicin binding by human erythrocytes. Antibiotiki i Chimioterapiya 39, No.9/10, 26–29 (in Russian)

3. Ataullakhanov, F.I., Batasheva, T.V., Vitvitsky, V.M. and Komarova, S.V. [1993] Effect of glutaraldehyde treatment on rubomycin and hemoglobin leakage from murine erythrocytes loaded with rubomycin. Biotekhnologiya, No. 2, 40–43 (in Russian)
4. Ataullakhanov, F.I., Kulikova, E.V. and Vitvitsky, V.M. [1994] Doxorubicin binding by human erythrocytes, in Carrier and Bioreactor Red Blood Cells for Drug Delivery and Targeting (DeLoach, J.R. and Way, J.L. eds.)., pp. 163–168. Elsevier Science Ltd, Oxford
5. Ataullakhanov, F.I., Vitvitsky, V.M., Kovaleva, V.L. and Mironova, S.B. [1992] Rubomycin loaded erythrocytes in the treatment of mouse tumor P388, in The Use of Resealed Erythrocytes as Carriers and Bioreactors (Magnani, M. and DeLoach, J.R. eds.)., pp. 209–213. Plenum Press, New York
6. Benjamin, R.S., Riggs, C.E. and Bachur, N.R. [1977] Plasma pharmacokinetics of adriamycin and its metabolites in humans with normal hepatic and renal function. Cancer Res. 37, 1416–1420
7. Cassiletti, P.A. and Katz, M.E. [1977] Chemotherapy for adult acute non lymphocytic leukemia with daunorubicin and cytosine arabinoside. Cancer Treat. Rep. 61, 1441–1445
8. DeFlora, A., Benatti, U., Guida, L. and Zocchi, E. [1986] Encapsulation of doxorubicin in human erythrocytes. Proc. Natl. Acad. Sci. USA. 83, 7029–7033
9. Gaudreault, R.C., Bellemare, B. and Lacroix, J. [1989] Erythrocyte membrane-bound daunorubicin as a delivery system in anticancer treatment. Anticancer Res. 9, 1201–1205
10. Gasparini, A., Tonetti, M., Astroff, B., Rowe, L., Satterfield, W., Schmidt, R. and DeLoach, J.R. [1992] Pharmacokinetics of doxorubicin loaded and glutaraldehyde treated erythrocytes in healthy and lymphoma bearing dogs, in The Use of Resealed Erythrocytes as Carriers and Bioreactors (Magnani, M. and DeLoach, J.R. eds.)., pp. 299–304. Plenum Press, New York
11. Kitao, T. and Hattori, K. [1980] Erythrocyte entrapment of daunomycin by amphotericin B without hemolysis. Cancer Res. 40, 1351–1353
12. Kitao, T., Hattori, K. and Takeshita, M. [1978] Agglutination of leukemic cells and daunomycin entrapped erythrocytes with lectin *in vitro* and *in vivo*. Experientia 34, 94–95
13. Lee, Y.-T.N., Chan, K.K., Harris, P.A. and Cohen, J.L. [1980] Distribution of adriamycin in cancer patients. Tissue uptakes, plasma concentration after IV and hepatic IA administration. Cancer 45, 2231–2239
14. Lefrak, E.A., Pitha, J., Rosenheim, S. and Gottlieb, J.A. [1973] A clinicopathologic analysis of adriamycin cardiotoxicity. Cancer 32, 302–314
15. Matherne, C.M., Satterfield, W.C., Gasparini, A., Tonetti, M., Astroff, A.B., Schmidt, R.D., Rowe, L.D. and DeLoach, J.R. [1994] Clinical efficacy and toxicity of doxorubicin encapsulated in glutaraldehyde-treated erythrocytes administered to dogs with lymphosarcoma. Am. J. Vet. Res. 55, 847–853
16. Rachman, A., Fumagalli, A., Barbieri, B., Schein, P. and Casazza, A.M. [1986] Antitumor and toxicity evaluation of free doxorubicin and doxorubicin entrapped in cardiolipin liposomes. Cancer Chemother. Pharmacol. 16, 22–27
17. Satterfield, W.C., Matherne, C.M., Clarke, M.S. and DeLoach, J.R. [1992] Clinical evaluation of glutaraldehyde-treated canine erythrocytesin normal dogs, in The Use of Resealed Erythrocytes as Carriers and Bioreactors (Magnani, M. and DeLoach, J.R. eds.)., pp. 319–324. Plenum Press, New York
18. Stenberg, C.P., Civin, C., Krischer, J., Culbert, S., Ragab, A., Ruymann, F.B., Ravindranath, J., Leventhal, B., Wilkinson, R. and Vietti, T.J. [1991] A comparison of induction and maintenance therapy for acute non-lymphocytic leukemia in childhood: results of a pediatric oncology group study. J. Clin. Oncol. 9, 247–288
19. Tonetti, M., Astroff, B., Satterfield, W., DeFlora, A., Benatti, U. and DeLoach, J.R. [1990] Construction and characterization of adriamycin-loaded canine red blood cells as a potential slow delivery system. Biotechnol. Appl. Biochem. 12, 621–629
20. Tonetti, M., Zocchi, E., Guida, Z., Polvani, C., Benatti, U., Biassoni, P., Romei, F., Guglielmi, A., Aschele, C., Sobrero, A. and DeFlora, A. [1992] Use of glutaraldehyde treated autologous human erythrocytes for hepatic targeting of doxorubicin, in The Use of Resealed Erythrocytes as Carriers and Bioreactors (Magnani, M. and DeLoach, J.R. eds.)., pp. 307–317. Plenum Press, New York
21. Zocchi, E., Tonetti, M., Polvani, C., Guida, Z., Benatti, U. and DeFlora, A. [1988] *In vivo* liver and lung targeting of adriamycin encapsulated in glutaraldehyde-treated murine erythrocytes. Biotechnol. Appl. Biochem. 10, 555–562
22. Zocchi, E., Tonetti, M., Polvani, C.,Guida, Z., Benatti, U. and DeFlora, A. [1989] Encapsulation of doxorubicin in liver-targeted erythrocytes increases the therapeutic index of the drug in murine metastatic model. Proc. Natl. Acad. Sci. USA. 86, 2040–2044

19

BINDING OF DAUNORUBICIN AND DOXORUBICIN TO ERYTHROCYTES TREATED WITH GLUTARALDEHYDE

Fazoil I. Ataullakhanov, Elena V. Kulikova, and Victor M. Vitvitsky

Scientific Center for Hematology of RAMS
125167 Moscow, Russia

1. ABSTRACT

Intact human erythrocytes can bind anthracycline antibiotics (daunorubicin and doxorubicin) during incubation in the isotonic medium containing the antibiotic. Bound antibiotics can be immobilized in the erythrocytes using glutaraldehyde treatment. It was found, however, that erythrocytes pretreated with glutaraldehyde can uptake daunorubicin and doxorubicin from the incubation medium and do it faster than untreated cells. The antibiotics are readily released from these erythrocytes in the antibiotic-free medium. Our findings provide evidence that immobilization of anthracycline antibiotics in the erythrocytes using glutaraldehyde treatment is connected with the chemical binding of the antibiotics to different erythrocyte components.

2. INTRODUCTION

Being very effective as antineoplastic drugs anthracycline antibiotics are highly toxic[7,12,14,15]. One of the ways to diminish toxic action of anthracycline antibiotics and to improve their therapeutic indexes is to use erythrocytes as drug carrier[1,9–11,18,19]. However, anthracycline antibiotics loaded into erythrocytes rapidly leak from the cell to the surrounding medium[3,8,10,16,18]. Anthracycline antibiotics can be immobilized in erythrocytes using glutaraldehyde treatment[3,9,16,18]. This treatment provides selective trapping of the treated erythrocytes by spleen, liver and lungs and, hence, results in targeting of entrapped drugs to these organs[18]. Doxorubicin-loaded and glutaraldehyde-treated erythrocytes have been shown to be more effective than the doxorubicin solution in prevention of experimental liver metastases in mice[19]. Daunorubicin-loaded and glutaraldehyde-treated erythrocytes have been shown to retain the antineoplastic activity after freezing and thawing[1]. This opens the possibility for storage of the beforehand prepared erythrocytes loaded with anthracycline antibiotics. Erythrocytes loaded with anthracycline antibiotics and then

Erythrocytes as Drug Carriers in Medicine, edited by Sprandel and Way
Plenum Press, New York, 1997

treated with glutaraldehyde seem to be extremely promising for therapeutic usage. First results of the clinical trial of doxorubicin-loaded and glutaraldehyde-treated erythrocytes in a patient with massive hepatic metastases and in dogs with lymphosarcoma were reported[13,17].

However, the mechanism responsible for anthracycline antibiotics immobilization in the glutaraldehyde-treated erythrocytes is not well understood. It is not clear if glutaraldehyde decreases the permeability of erythrocyte membrane to anthracycline antibiotics or it chemically binds anthracycline antibiotics to different erythrocyte components. The latter seems more plausible because glutaraldehyde is able to form chemical bonds between substances containing amino groups[6]. Molecules of anthracycline antibiotics contain one amino group; therefore, they can form chemical bonds via glutaraldehyde to different amino-group-containing erythrocyte components. To understand *in vivo* functioning of drug carrier erythrocytes in full detail, it is necessary to know the exact mechanism of glutaraldehyde-mediated immobilization of anthracycline antibiotics in these cells.

In this work, we studied the ability of glutaraldehyde-treated human erythrocytes (GTE) to bind daunorubicin and doxorubicin. It was shown earlier that native erythrocytes are able to bind these antibiotics in a reversible manner[2–5,16,17]. We expected that, if glutaraldehyde treatment decreases the permeability of erythrocyte membrane to anthracycline antibiotics, it would decrease or abolish binding of these antibiotics to erythrocytes.

3. MATERIALS AND METHODS

Pharmaceutic preparation of daunorubicin (rubomycin hydrochloride) was from FAO Ferein (Mosmedpreparaty, Moscow, Russia). Doxorubicin was used as adriablastin, commercially available from Farmitalia Carlo Erba (Montedison Group, Italy). Glutaraldehyde (70% aqueous solution) was from Serva, (Germany).

Erythrocytes were isolated from preserved donor blood by centrifugation, then washed two times by resuspension in a double volume of glucose containing phosphate buffered saline (GPBS) and following centrifugation at 1500g for 10 min. Washed erythrocytes were split into two portions. One portion of erythrocytes was used as control and the other was treated with glutaraldehyde. Control and glutaraldehide-treated packed erythrocytes were brought to the desirable temperature and resuspended to hematocrit about 50% in the solution of daunorubicin (or doxorubicin) in GPBS maintained at the same temperature. The pH values of daunorubicin and doxorubicin solutions were 7.4 and 7.0, respectively. The prepared suspensions of control erythrocytes or GTE (hematocrit 50%) were incubated at constant temperature and periodic stirring. Concentrations of anthracycline antibiotics in the incubation medium were measured during the incubation to evaluate binding of antibiotics to erythrocytes. The release of anthracycline antibiotics was studied using GTE which were loaded with the antibiotic by a 30-min incubation in the antibiotic-containing medium at 24°C. Then suspension was centrifugated at 1500g for 3 min, supernatant was discarded and packed GTE were resuspended in an equal volume of GPBS to hematocrit 50%. In order to evaluate the antibiotic release from the GTE, its concentration in the incubation medium was measured 5 min after the resuspension.

Glutaraldehyde treatment procedure was based on the earlier described method[1,3,16]. Erythrocytes were mixed with an equal volume of 0.35% glutaraldehyde solution in GPBS and the mixture was incubated at room temperature for 15 min. Erythrocytes then were washed four times by resuspension in 10 volumes of GPBS followed by centrifugation at

1500g for 3 min. GPBS containing 10 mM of glycine was used for the first washing in order to eliminate unreacted glutaraldehyde.

To determine concentrations of daunorubicin or doxorubicin chloroform extracts were prepared from supernatants obtained by centrifugation of samples of the erythrocyte suspension as it was described earlier[2–4]. Concentrations of antibiotics in the chloroform extracts were determined spectrophotometrically. To this end, optical density of chloroform extracts were measured in 1 cm quartz cells using pure chloroform as a blank. Measurements were made at the wavelength of the corresponding maximum of antibiotic visible spectrum (485 nm for doxorubicin and 500 nm for daunorubicin). For calibration of the measurements standard solutions of daunorubicin or doxorubicin in chloroform were used.

4. RESULTS

GTE retain their ability to bind anthracycline antibiotics. Moreover, compared with untreated erythrocytes, GTE bind anthracycline antibiotics faster. Figure 1 shows the uptake of daunorubicin from the incubation medium by GTE versus untreated erythrocytes. These results were obtained on erythrocytes of five different donors. Under our experimental conditions, untreated erythrocytes bind about 70% of daunorubicin from the medium within 30 min, in agreement with the data reported earlier[2,3,5], whereas GTE uptake about 85% of daunorubicin within only 5 min. In contrast to untreated cells[2,5], GTE seem

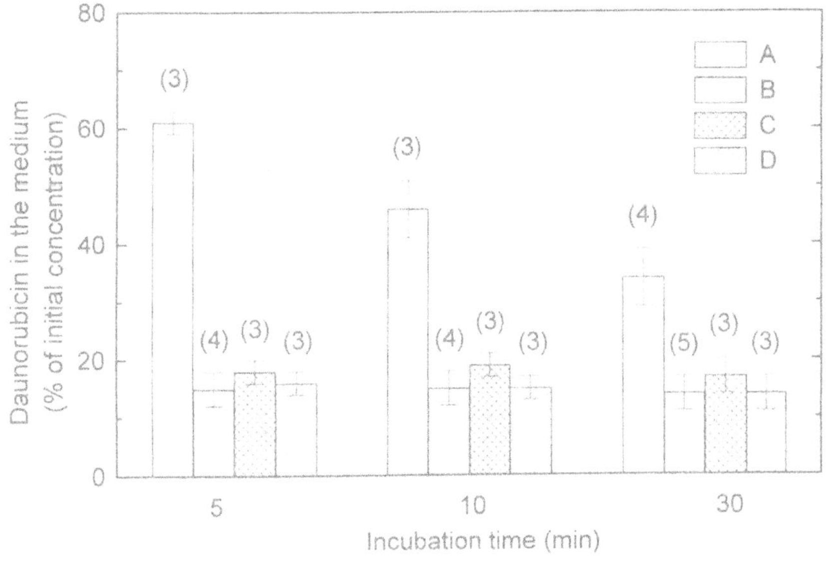

Figure 1. Binding of daunorubicin to glutaraldehyde-treated erythrocytes (GTE). (A) control (untreated) erythrocytes, 24°C, initial daunorubicin concentration in the medium, 0.81±0.02 mg/ml; (B) GTE, 24°C, initial daunorubicin concentration in the medium, 1.00±0.02 mg/ml; (C) GTE, 24°C, initial daunorubicin concentration in the medium, 3.00±0.04 mg/ml; (D) GTE, 4°C, initial daunorubicin concentration in the medium, 1.00±0.02 mg/ml. Number of experiments, each performed on erythrocytes of one individual donor, are indicated in parentheses. In total, erythrocytes of five donors were used.

to bind daunorubicin independently of the initial antibiotic concentration and low temperature.

Doxorubicin showed a similar pattern of binding to GTE. Figure 2 demonstrates the results of a representative experiment arbitrarily chosen of two. Note that GTE bind doxorubicin faster than untreated cells. However, the effect is less pronounced than that observed with daunorubicin.

Anthracycline antibiotics bound to GTE are partially released from the erythrocytes after replacement of the incubation medium by fresh, antibiotic free solution. This release is completed within about 5 min after the replacement, and since then antibiotic concentration in the medium remains almost unchanged for at least an hour. The results of two separate experiments that demonstrate the release of daunorubicin from erythrocytes, treated with glutaraldehyde and then loaded with daunorubicin, are presented in Table 1. After each replacement of the incubation medium, significant amounts of daunorubicin appear in the medium due to its release from the GTE.

5. DISCUSSION

Our results suggest that treatment of erythrocytes with glutaraldehyde as such does not abolish or decrease their ability to bind anthracycline antibiotics. Consequently, one may conclude that glutaraldehyde treatment does not decrease the permeability of erythrocyte membrane to these antibiotics. Compared with untreated erythrocytes, GTE uptake anthracycline antibiotics more rapidly. Anthracycline antibiotics are amphifillic; therefore, it is plausible to suggest that glutaraldehyde treatment of erythrocytes diminishes the

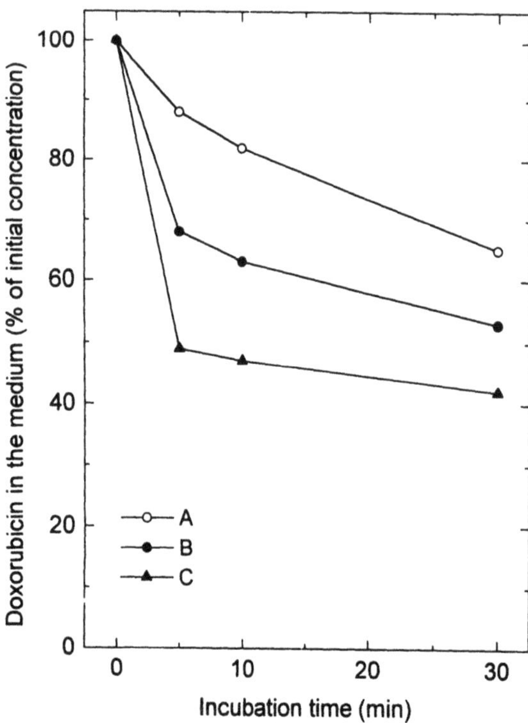

Figure 2. Binding of doxorubicin to glutaraldehyde-treated erythrocytes (GTE) at 18°C. (A) control (untreated) erythrocytes, initial doxorubicin concentration in the medium, 0.17 mg/ml; (B) GTE, initial doxorubicin concentration in the medium, 0.19 mg/ml; (C) GTE, initial doxorubicin concentration in the medium, 0.57 mg/ml.

Table 1. Release of daunorubicin from glutaraldehyde-treated human erythrocytes (GTE) in a series of successive replacement of the incubation medium. GTE were previously loaded with daunorubicin by incubation at 24°C for 30 min in the daunorubicin containing medium (hematocrit, 50%). The initial concentration of daunorubicin in the medium was 1 mg/ml

	Medium daunorubicin (mg/ml)	
Replacement of the medium	Exp. 1	Exp. 2
1-st	0.087	0.11
2-nd	0.068	0.074
3-rd	0.060	0.046

amount of the polar groups on the cell surface and facilitates the interaction between anthracycline antibiotics and hydrophobic lipid compartment within the cell membrane.

Binding of anthracycline antibiotics by erythrocytes pretreated with glutaraldehyde is reversible. The finding that erythrocytes treated with glutaraldehyde and then loaded with daunorubicin rapidly release daunorubicin after replacement of the incubation medium (Table 1) supports this suggestion. In a series of successive replacements of the incubation medium, each replacement resulted in the substantial appearance of daunorubicin in the medium. This finding provides evidence that we observed the release of daunorubicin rather than the contamination of the packed cells by the remaining incubation medium. By contrast, there is no similar leakage of the antibiotics from those erythrocytes that were first loaded with anthracycline antibiotics and then treated with glutaraldehyde[3,16,18]. It is conceivable that glutaraldehyde treatment of erythrocytes loaded with anthracycline antibiotics results in the irreversible chemical binding of the antibiotics to different erythrocyte components.

Specific activities, toxicities, and therapeutic indexes of various anthracycline antibiotics are very different in spite of the apparent slight differences in their chemical structures. Therefore, it is plausible that modification of the structure of anthracycline antibiotics caused by their immobilization within erythrocytes via glutaraldehyde could also modify properties of the original drugs. Moreover, such a modification may significantly depend on details of the glutaraldehyde treatment procedure. Modification of the drug during the glutaraldehyde treatment may explain the occurrence of some unexpected side effects caused by administration of doxorubicin-loaded and glutaraldehyde-treated erythrocytes[13,17]. It is our opinion, however, that the results obtained do not exclude the possibility for the use of erythrocytes as carriers of anthracycline antibiotics. First of all, the preparation of anthracycline antibiotic carrier erythrocytes do not necessarily imply the treatment with glutaraldehyde. Daunorubicin loaded erythrocytes prepared without glutaraldehyde treatment were shown to increase the specific activity[10,11] and decrease toxicity[1] of daunorubicin. Next, strict standardization of the glutaraldrhyde treatment procedure can unify glutaraldehyde treated carrier erythrocytes and, hence, decrease the probability of unexpected side effects of their usage.

6. REFERENCES

1. Ataullakhanov, F.I., Batasheva, T.V., Bukhman, V.M., Komarova, S.V., Oreshkina, T.D. and Vitvitsky, V.M. [1994] Treatment of Rausher virus induced murine erythroblastic leukemia with rubomycin loaded erythro-

cytes, in Carrier and Bioreactor Red Blood Cells for Drug Delivery and Targeting (DeLoach, J.R. and Way, J.L. eds.)., pp. 177–183. Elsevier Science Ltd, Oxford

2. Ataullakhanov, F.I., Batasheva, T.V. and Vitvitsky, V.M. [1994] Influence of temperature, daunorubicin concentration and suspension hematocrit on daunorubicin binding by human erythrocytes. Antibiotiki i Chimioterapiya 39, No. 9/10, 26–29 (in Russian)
3. Ataullakhanov, F.I., Batasheva, T.V., Vitvitsky, V.M. and Komarova, S.V. [1993] Effect of glutaraldehyde treatment on rubomycin and hemoglobin leakage from murine erythrocytes loaded with rubomycin. Biotekhnologiya No. 2, 40–43 (in Russian)
4. Ataullakhanov,F.I., Kulikova, E.V. and Vitvitsky, V.M. [1994] Doxorubicin binding by human erythrocytes, in Carrier and Bioreactor Red Blood Cells for Drug Delivery and Targeting (DeLoach, J.R. and Way, J.L. eds.)., pp. 163–168. Elsevier Science Ltd, Oxford
5. Ataullakhanov, F.I., Vitvitsky, V.M., Kovaleva, V.L. and Mironova, S.B. [1992] Rubomycin loaded erythrocytes in the treatment of mouse tumor P388, in The Use of Resealed Erythrocytes as Carriers and Bioreactors (Magnani, M. and DeLoach, J.R. eds.)., pp. 209–213. Plenum Press, New York
6. Avrameas, S. and Ternynck, T. [1969] The cross-linking of proteins with glutaraldehyde and its use for the preparation of immunosorbents. Immunochemistry 6, 53–66
7. Cassiletti, P.A. and Katz, M.E. [1977] Chemotherapy for adult acute non lymphocytic leukemia with daunorubicin and cytosine arabinoside. Cancer Treat. Rep. 61, 1441–1445
8. DeFlora, A., Benatti, U., Guida, L. and Zocchi, E. [1986] Encapsulation of doxorubicin in human erythrocytes. Proc. Natl. Acad. Sci. USA. 83, 7029–7033
9. Gaudreault, R.C., Bellemare, B. and Lacroix, J. [1989] Erythrocyte membrane-bound daunorubicin as a delivery system in anticancer treatment. Anticancer Res. 9, 1201–1205
10. Kitao, T. and Hattori, K. [1980] Erythrocyte entrapment of daunomycin by amphotericin B without hemolysis. Cancer Res. 40, 1351–1353
11. Kitao, T., Hattori, K. and Takeshita, M. [1978] Agglutination of leukemic cells and daunomycin entrapped erythrocytes with lectin *in vitro* and *in vivo*. Experientia 34, 94–95
12. Lefrak, E.A., Pitha, J., Rosenheim, S. and Gottlieb, J.A. [1973] A clinicopathologic analysis of adriamycin cardiotoxicity. Cancer 32, 302–314
13. Matherne, C.M., Satterfield, W.C., Gasparini, A., Tonetti, M., Astroff, A.B., Schmidt, R.D., Rowe, L.D. and DeLoach, J.R. [1994] Clinical efficacy and toxicity of doxorubicin encapsulated in glutaraldehyde-treated erythrocytes administered to dogs with lymphosarcoma. Am. J. Vet. Res. 55, 847–853
14. Rachman, A., Fumagalli, A., Barbieri, B., Schein, P. and Casazza, A.M. [1986] Antitumor and toxicity evaluation of free doxorubicin and doxorubicin entrapped in cardiolipin liposomes. Cancer Chemother. Pharmacol. 16, 22–27
15. Stenberg, C.P., Civin, C., Krischer, J., Culbert, S., Ragab, A., Ruymann, F.B., Ravindranath, J., Leventhal, B., Wilkinson, R. and Vietti, T.J. [1991] A comparison of induction and maintenance therapy for acute non-lymphocytic leukemia in childhood: results of a pediatric oncology group study. J. Clin. Oncol. 9, 247–288
16. Tonetti, M., Astroff, B., Satterfield, W., DeFlora, A., Benatti, U. and DeLoach, J.R. [1990] Construction and characterization of adriamycin-loaded canine red blood cells as a potential slow delivery system. Biotechnol. Appl. Biochem. 12, 621–629
17. Tonetti, M., Zocchi, E., Guida, Z., Polvani, C., Benatti, U., Biassoni, P., Romei, F., Guglielmi, A., Aschele, C. Sobrero, A. and DeFlora, A. [1992] Use of glutaraldehyde treated autologous human erythrocytes for hepatic targeting of doxorubicin, in The Use of Resealed Erythrocytes as Carriers and Bioreactors (Magnani, M. and DeLoach, J.R. eds.)., pp. 307–317. Plenum Press, New York
18. Zocchi, E., Tonetti, M., Polvani, C., Guida, Z., Benatti, U. and DeFlora, A. [1988] *In vivo* liver and lung targeting of adriamycin encapsulated in glutaraldehyde-treated murine erythrocytes. Biotechnol. Appl. Biochem. 10, 555–562
19. Zocchi, E., Tonetti, M., Polvani, C.,Guida, Z., Benatti, U. and DeFlora, A. [1989] Encapsulation of doxorubicin in liver-targeted erythrocytes increases the therapeutic index of the drug in murine metastatic model. Proc. Natl. Acad. Sci. USA. 86, 2040–2044

INDEX

GPSR Compliance
The European Union's (EU) General Product Safety Regulation (GPSR) is a set of rules that requires consumer products to be safe and our obligations to ensure this.

If you have any concerns about our products, you can contact us on

ProductSafety@springernature.com

In case Publisher is established outside the EU, the EU authorized representative is:

Springer Nature Customer Service Center GmbH
Europaplatz 3
69115 Heidelberg, Germany

www.ingramcontent.com/pod-product-compliance
Ingram Content Group UK Ltd.
Pitfield, Milton Keynes, MK11 3LW, UK
UKHW051130260726
13967UKWH00010B/2959

* 9 7 8 1 4 8 9 9 0 0 4 5 6 *